This book is the gold standard; in its contribution to our understanding of pathological lying, nothing else compares. Curtis and Hart have brought order to a confused, disorganized, but deeply significant topic. Their research is cutting-edge, and their recommendations for the assessment and diagnosis of pathological lying are impressively justified and badly needed.

—BELLA DePAULO, PhD, ACADEMIC AFFILIATE, DEPARTMENT OF PSYCHOLOGICAL AND BRAIN SCIENCES, UNIVERSITY OF CALIFORNIA, SANTA BARBARA, SANTA BARBARA, CA, UNITED STATES

The most frequent question we deception researchers are asked is, "What about pathological liars?" Now we can answer, "Buy this book." It fills a gap in the literature by providing a comprehensive overview of theory, research, and clinical practice related to pathological lying, and is written in a very accessible style.

—ALDERT VRIJ, PhD, PROFESSOR OF APPLIED SOCIAL PSYCHOLOGY, DEPARTMENT OF PSYCHOLOGY, UNIVERSITY OF PORTSMOUTH, PORTSMOUTH, HANTS, ENGLAND

By parsing pathological lying from everyday normative and prolific lying, Curtis and Hart make a valuable contribution to both clinical psychology and the study of deception. Not only do they build the case for pathological lying as a distinct diagnosis that is more than just the symptom of other pathologies, but they also help us to understand that not everyone who tells a lot of lies is suffering from a mental disorder. This book will go a long way toward correcting the frequent and casual misuse of the term "pathological liar."

—KIM SEROTA, PhD, DECEPTION SCHOLAR AND LECTURER, DEPARTMENT OF MANAGEMENT AND MARKETING, OAKLAND UNIVERSITY, ROCHESTER, MI, UNITED STATES

Curtis and Hart provide the much-needed definitive treatise on pathological lying. They have changed how I understand pathological lying. I recommend their book to everyone interested in the topic.

—TIMOTHY R. LEVINE, PhD, AUTHOR OF *DUPED: TRUTH-DEFAULT THEORY AND THE SOCIAL SCIENCE OF LYING AND DECEPTION*

Following an outstanding review of the literature, the authors use case histories and examples, historical and current, to bring the concept of pathological lying to life. This scholarly but easy-to-read work extends the forceful argument for recognizing pathological lying as a diagnostic entity in the *DSM*.

—CHARLES C. DIKE, MD, MPH, DISTINGUISHED FELLOW, AMERICAN PSYCHIATRIC ASSOCIATION; FELLOW, ROYAL COLLEGE OF PSYCHIATRISTS OF ENGLAND; ASSOCIATE PROFESSOR OF PSYCHIATRY AND CO-DIRECTOR, LAW AND PSYCHIATRY DIVISION, YALE UNIVERSITY SCHOOL OF MEDICINE, NEW HAVEN, CT, UNITED STATES

Until now, our understanding of the pathological liar has been fragmented, confusing, and obscured by stigma. Finally, the picture is clearer! Curtis and Hart bring all the pieces of the puzzle together to provide an engaging book that draws on scientific evidence to help us understand the pathological liar—what makes them lie and approaches to reducing their lying and the negative impact on close personal relationships.

—VICTORIA TALWAR, PhD, AUTHOR OF *THE TRUTH ABOUT LYING: TEACHING HONESTY TO CHILDREN AT EVERY AGE AND STAGE*; PROFESSOR AND CHAIR, DEPARTMENT OF EDUCATIONAL AND COUNSELLING PSYCHOLOGY, McGILL UNIVERSITY, MONTREAL, QC, CANADA

PATHOLOGICAL
LYING

PATHOLOGICAL
LYING

THEORY, RESEARCH, AND PRACTICE

DREW A. CURTIS AND
CHRISTIAN L. HART

 AMERICAN PSYCHOLOGICAL ASSOCIATION

Published by
American Psychological Association
750 First Street, NE
Washington, DC 20002
https://www.apa.org

Order Department
https://www.apa.org/pubs/books
order@apa.org

In the U.K., Europe, Africa, and the Middle East, copies may be ordered from Eurospan
https://www.eurospanbookstore.com/apa
info@eurospangroup.com

Typeset in Minion by Circle Graphics, Inc., Reisterstown, MD

Printer: Gasch Printing, Odenton, MD
Cover Designer: Mark Karis

Library of Congress Cataloging-in-Publication Data

Names: Curtis, Drew A., author. | Hart, Christian L., author.
Title: Pathological lying : theory, research, and practice / by Drew A. Curtis
    and Christian L. Hart.
Description: Washington : American Psychological Association, [2023] |
    Includes bibliographical references and index.
Identifiers: LCCN 2022003010 (print) | LCCN 2022003011 (ebook) |
    ISBN 9781433836220 (paperback) | ISBN 9781433835636 (ebook)
Subjects: LCSH: Deception. | Mythomania. | Psychology, Pathological. |
    Truthfulness and falsehood.
Classification: LCC RC569.5.D44 C76 2023 (print) | LCC RC569.5.D44
    (ebook) | DDC 616.85/84--dc23/eng/20220215
LC record available at https://lccn.loc.gov/2022003010
LC ebook record available at https://lccn.loc.gov/2022003011

https://doi.org/10.1037/0000305-000

Printed in the United States of America

10 9 8 7 6 5 4 3 2 1

Contents

CONTENTS

Preface

When things puzzle or confuse us, or are not quickly understood, it often seems easier to look away and carry on with life. Providing a catch-all term of "crazy" may assist with labeling a phenomenon and moving on. To that notion, it is a great disservice with potentially grave consequences for the individuals who struggle. A more effortful—and arguably rewarding—path is to lean in and seek understanding. Our compassion for those suffering and our desire to shed light on a neglected phenomenon fueled this attempt to consolidate a scattered literature on pathological lying and to synthesize a more complete understanding of the phenomenon.

For more than a century, pathological lying has been recognized and discussed among various professionals. In fact, pathological lying has carried many names, including pseudologia phantastica, habitual lying, compulsive lying, morbid lying, and mythomania. Yet the zeitgeist appears to have left many of these writings on pathological lying in the past or scattered among the literature. Today, we find that "pathological lying" is a term that is more commonplace or easily recognized among popular culture, though it is not fully understood. Even so, pathological lying has not been formally recognized as a psychological disorder within diagnostic systems. Simply, a person who struggles with pathological lying is unable to receive a diagnosis or suitable treatment for their problematic behavior.

GOALS

One of our goals was to address this concern by synthesizing research, applying theory, and reporting the current scientific findings on pathological lying, with the intent to advance a more comprehensive understanding. This book addresses the hole within the literature by establishing the theoretical and empirical foundations for pathological lying by integrating deception research within the clinical context. We drew from recent deception frequency research and contemporary theories and standards of psychopathology to examine pathological lying. Our theory-driven research has corroborated the existence of pathological lying and helped set parameters and definitions to more clearly discuss and study pathological lying.

We hope that our attempts to unify nomenclature and provide a conceptual framework for pathological lying will stimulate research and equip practitioners to better assess, diagnose, and treat pathological lying. Researchers and clinicians will be able to identify a group of people who are categorically distinct in telling lies that are pathological and problematic for the person. By providing an understanding of normative deception, a definition of pathological lying, theory-driven research findings, etiological markers, assessment profiles, case studies, and clinicians' perceptions and experiences, we hope that researchers and clinicians will be positioned to understand and recognize some of the complexities of pathological lying.

Along these lines, we hope that this work will facilitate the recognition of pathological lying as a distinct diagnostic entity for psychiatry and psychology. In doing so, those who suffer from pathological lying may be able to more easily seek out help and treatment from licensed mental health practitioners. We have provided a framework and suggested measures as well as diagnostic criteria to assist practitioners in clinical assessment. Our hope is that this book will be a clinical reference for academicians who train mental health practitioners, specifically in dealing with pathological lying within the psychotherapeutic context. Further, we hope that these markers will facilitate clinical research related to the treatment of pathological lying.

A broad social goal is to help the general public better understand pathological lying. Our hope is that the general public may see that pathological liars are not cold, calculated, and malicious people who are out to undermine everyone they come in contact with but rather that they are often suffering from their behavior and unable to change on their own. Thus, a deeper understanding of pathological lying may challenge myths and misconceptions and reduce stigma.

STRUCTURE

The first chapter presents an overview of pathological lying, some of the historical accounts of pathological lying, and previous definitions and offers a current definition of pathological lying. The second and third chapters review the various aspects of deception and lying and unpack characteristics of people who tend to tell excessive lies. The fourth chapter presents historical accounts of pathological lying and sets the stage for the current research related to pathological lying, which is found in the fifth chapter. The sixth chapter examines aspects of lying within the psychotherapeutic contexts, giving attention to the occurrence of pathological lying in psychotherapy. The last three chapters relate to the clinical process of assessment, diagnosis, and treatment of pathological lying. In the final chapter, we address some of the limitations, challenges, and areas for future research on pathological lying.

CASES

We hold compassion and concern for individuals who have expressed difficulties from pathological lying. Within this book, we discuss various people who have been identified in the literature as pathological liars, who have self-identified as pathological liars, or who have demonstrated features related to pathological lying. We want to respect those individuals who have shared their struggles and preserve their confidentiality and privacy as best we can. Unless the information has been previously published, we altered some features and characteristics of the individual cases that we reference within this book. We withheld individuals' names to protect their identities. In some cases, we reported a collection of accounts from various individuals. Our goal of sharing these examples and cases is to facilitate understanding about pathological lying and to promote research and practice that better helps these individuals.

Acknowledgments

We thank our families for their unending patience, love, and support throughout this book project. We also thank Timothy R. Levine, Kim B. Serota, and Bella M. DePaulo for the inspiration they offered in several areas of this book. Additionally, we want to extend our gratitude to the anonymous reviewers who were encouraging and provided useful feedback. Lastly, we thank Emily Ekle, Krissy Jones, and all the American Psychological Association team who have supported this idea and worked diligently on this text.

PATHOLOGICAL
LYING

Pathological Lying: An Overview

A severe snowstorm had blanketed the countryside of Poland during the travels of Baron Munchausen. Weary, he decided to cease travel for a night's rest. He tied his horse to some pointed object that resembled a tree stump emerging out from the snow, secured his firearms under his arms, and soundly fell fast asleep in the snow. When the Baron woke, he was lying in a village churchyard, and his horse was hanging from the weather-cock of the steeple. The deep snow had melted overnight, leaving the horse caught on the steeple and the Baron lying on the ground. Without much deliberation, the Baron quickly fired a shot at his horse's bridle, which successfully freed his equine companion (Raspe, 2013). Unique stories, such as the adventures of Baron Munchausen, fascinate us. However, exaggerated stories, if told as truths, lead to skepticism and distrust. People do not like liars.

https://doi.org/10.1037/0000305-001
Pathological Lying: Theory, Research, and Practice, by D. A. Curtis and C. L. Hart

People often have a fascination with abnormal behaviors and rare circumstances, wanting a glimpse, but not wanting to get too close. The disheveled man on the street who talks to his hallucinations garners attention from the passersby. The child with autism who is having a tantrum in a store draws looks from other shoppers. Movies and shows that document a person's strange addictions such as eating drywall or hoarding broken appliances get viewer interest. Psychopathology has long captivated human curiosity, and pathological lying is no different.

At the same time, people tend to fear the unknown. The onlookers keep a safe distance when sneaking a peek at the man who aberrantly speaks to air. The shoppers steal a glance at the child's screaming and flailing without getting noticed by the child's parent. Movies and shows offer us the safety of watching other people's atypical behavior from the safety of a screen and the comfort of our couch.

When we consider the pathological liar, the same pattern appears to emerge. Those people who deign to flaunt the norms of honesty are spectacles that grip us and mesmerize us. They leave us fascinated. As much as pathological liars hold our attention, we also tend to resist affiliating with those who regularly lie to us. Liars are unreliable, disloyal, and even dangerous. They warp the very foundation of human relationships—trust.

The concept of pathological lying is widespread, and the term is foreign to few. Yet shockingly, the scientific community has made little effort or progress toward understanding pathological liars. Can we use the tool of science to understand pathological lying? When most people consider the pathological liar, they often assume the dishonesty is rooted in pure wickedness or think of pathological liars as monsters who seek to bring havoc everywhere. But might extreme forms of lying actually be symptoms of mental illness? Could it be that people who lie pathologically are actually the ones who suffer most from their lies? Like other forms of mental illness, could we not, perhaps, assess, diagnose, and treat pathological lying? Our goal has been to more closely examine pathological lying and to offer scientific advances in this area. Ultimately, we hope to illuminate and understand the world of the pathological liar, shedding light on the causal mechanisms of their disordered prevarications and proposing approaches that may aid in reducing their lying to the benefit of the liars and the people around them.

Evidence of lying can be found in written records throughout world history. Historical, cultural, and religious documentation of lying and liars is robust and unequivocal. Lies and liars are viewed negatively. The Bible addresses lies and deceit throughout scripture. Within the first book of the Bible, Genesis, the serpent deceives Eve by telling her that it is acceptable to eat the fruit that God had commanded them not to eat (Genesis 3:1, English Standard Version). The act of lying as an abomination and unwise is recorded throughout the Bible. Satan is referred to as the Father of Lies (John 8:44, English Standard Version). In addition to religious texts, ancient Greek philosophers such as Aristotle discussed the ethics and virtues of being honest and truthful (Aristotle, 1941a). Lying was not viewed as virtuous. Other ancient, nonreligious texts, such as the Code of Hammurabi, portrayed liars as deserving of death (L. W. King, 2008). In general, liars are stereotypically painted as "cold and exploitative" (DePaulo et al., 2004, p. 147). Being called a liar can even be considered a "mortal insult" (Bok, 1999, p. 38). In fact, of 555 personality trait words, the word *liar* falls at the bottom, as the least liked trait (N. H. Anderson, 1968). Thus, people across cultures and throughout time have asserted that lying and liars are morally reprehensible, negative, bad, and sinful.

A great danger exists for the person who lies excessively—not only because of the potential harm from the lies but because of the resignation of their credibility and reliability. Most people do not expect complete and utter honesty from others. Leniency is granted to people who tell occasional lies, especially when those lies are of little significance, when the lies only serve "social niceties" and are intended to benefit others. People who occasionally lie are mostly honest, which provides some certainty and about their trustworthiness when interacting with them. Most of us operate within cultures where most people can be trusted at their word most of the time. The assumption that most people are honest most of the time aligns with reality; Levine (2014b, 2020) referred to this expectation of truthfulness as "truth-default."

The very fabric of human society and interpersonal exchanges hinges on an honesty assumption, or a truth default. It would be difficult if not nearly impossible to accomplish any feat if it required individuals to sift through all information to ascertain which information was reliable. If honesty was always in question, business transactions would grind to a halt, relationships would bog down in endless verifications of sentiments, and interpersonal bonds would strain under questions of loyalty. In application, the practice of medicine requires an assumption of accurate and reliable reporting of symptoms. Similarly, the practice of psychotherapy requires the same assumptions. For example, one specific case of a patient who fabricated an entire therapeutic persona ultimately ended in a waste of time and resources, with no psychotherapeutic benefit and the patient potentially taking away the opportunity for the practitioner to help another individual (Grzegorek, 2011).

The concern of trustworthiness and being a reliable source of information was at the center of Kant's (1797/1996) argument of individuals' duties to be honest. Kant believed people should strive for honesty in all situations. It has been argued that Kant has the strongest position on the prohibition against lying (Bok, 1999). The idea of radical honesty in which one is always truthful provides a complete sense of consistency for oneself and for others. However, it is obvious that humanity does not adhere to Kant's precept, as most, if not all, humans lie. It is worth noting that while most people have lied, most people do not lie often (Curtis & Hart, 2020a; Curtis et al., 2021; Serota & Levine, 2015; Serota et al., 2010). Thus, the reliance on a truth bias largely dovetails with how the world operates, in that most people can be relied on to be honest most of the time. Generally, this way of thinking offers consistency and cognitive efficiency. However scarce lying is, it does still occur with predictable regularity, carrying with it enormous societal consequences.

DECEPTION AND LYING

The vested interest in understanding how to discern the veracity of others' statements has led to a plethora of research on the topic of deception. Research on liars and lie detection has grown significantly over the past 60 years (see McGlone & Knapp, 2019). The study of deception is multidisciplinary, with findings emerging from anthropology, art, biology, botany, communication, economics, entomology, history, journalism, law, management, mathematics, media studies, medicine, psychiatry, philosophy, physics, psychology, political science, public policy, advertising, sociology, religion, sociology, and zoology (see McGlone & Knapp, 2019). Interest in deception and its detection has prompted government agencies, corporations, and others to fund a substantial body of deception research. More than $1 million from the U.S. Federal Bureau of Investigations and Department of Defense has been issued to fund projects from some of the leading experts in deception. These agencies have a special interest in detecting deception, but so does the general public. Relationally, people are interested to know whether a significant other is secretly interested in another person, a child has been using illicit drugs, a parent has been forthcoming about finances, or a friend is using you for selfish gain. It is evident that everyday people, professionals, and agencies are curious to understand deception and want to learn how to better detect it.

Before wading too deep into a discussion about lying, it is important to first provide a basic definition of the phenomenon. Regarding deception, several prominent scholars have put forth a variety of definitions, with each building on or making some subtle and important clarifications. Definitions are discussed in more detail in the next chapter. The definition we use for deception is from Vrij (2000): *lying* is "a successful or unsuccessful deliberate attempt, without forewarning, to create in another a belief which the communicator considers to be untrue" (p. 6). Building on Vrij, Hart (2019) suggested that lying is different from deception and defined it as "a successful or unsuccessful deliberate manipulation of language, without forewarning, to create in another a belief which the communicator considers to be untrue."

Scholars have traditionally discussed deception in two categorical dimensions: ethics and normativity. The majority of deception literature has discussed the normative aspects of lying, such as the prevalence and frequency of lying within the general population (see Levine, 2014a, 2020; Vrij, 2008). Even the most heavily researched and funded aspect of deception, its detection, tends to focus on detecting deception from the perspective of the typical person (Granhag et al., 2015). In addition to the normative aspects of lying, there has been ample debate about deception and whether its use is ethical (e.g., Baumrind, 1985; Bok, 1999; Curtis et al., 2020; Curtis & Kelley, 2020b; Levine & Schweitzer, 2014; 2015; Sade, 2012; Tavaglione & Hurst, 2012). Much less has been written about the pathology of lying. Of the literature that has discussed pathological aspects of lying, it has largely remained fragmented or has not been discussed much, or at all, in other deception literature. The goal of this book is to focus on further understanding the pathological aspects of lying and synthesizing the existing literature in this area.

A LIAR

He does not answer questions, or gives evasive answers; he speaks nonsense, rubs the great toe along the ground; and shivers; his face is discolored; he rubs the roots of his hair with his fingers.—Description of a liar, 900 BC. (Global Deception Research Team, 2006, p. 60)

The label of *liar* has been used throughout history and within deception research but has rarely been the object of study (Curtis, 2021b). Liar is often descriptive of another person and is rarely used to describe one's own behaviors or traits (Curtis, 2021b). People generally like to think of themselves as good people. Using the term *liar* for one's own behaviors would threaten the consistency of self-image or, in other words, would cause cognitive dissonance or a discrepant perspective (Bok, 1999; Festinger, 1957). It is intuitive that a person would likely avoid labeling themselves as a liar to preserve their self-concept as a good, honest, and upright person.

The use of the label *liar* raises the question of when we should label someone so. Elsewhere, we have considered whether the label should be applied to anyone who has ever lied, based on the relative frequency with which people lie, based on the consequences of the lies, or the situational contexts in which lies occur (Curtis, 2021b; Hart & Curtis, in press). If we classify liars based on whether a person has ever lied, then virtually every person over age 3 years old would be a liar, as that is the approximate age in development where lying is evidenced (Sodian, 1991; Talwar & Lee, 2002b). If being a liar is based on the relative frequency with which people tell lies, then most people, although having lied, do not lie often (Curtis & Hart, 2020a; Serota et al., 2010; Serota & Levine, 2015). Thus, only high-frequency liars earn the label. If being a liar is based on the harm resulting from the lie, then the application of the label would be a nuanced calculation involving all parties that were affected. People tend to label others more as a liar when a lie is judged to be more serious (Curtis, 2021b). Going further, the tendency to call others a liar is also based on the type of lie told, where others who tell fabrications are judged more as liars than those who tell white lies or exaggerations (Curtis, 2021b). Pragmatically, people are labeled liars when they lie (Curtis, 2021b).

One of the potential dangers of labeling others as liars is the negative attitudes or stigma that could stem from such labels. People tend to hold more negative attitudes toward others who are thought to be liars (Curtis, 2021b; Curtis & Hart, 2015). However, this is largely due, as previously mentioned, to the influence of anecdotal experiences and the historical stereotype of liars. The potential concern of labeling others as pathological liars is also worth consideration (Curtis & Hart, 2020a). It is unclear, and no research has been conducted to our knowledge, whether people may harbor negative attitudes toward pathological liars based on the label itself or based on the concern of potentially being lied to by the person. We encourage research in this vein, to explore social cognitions and perceptions of pathological liars. It has been argued that stigma resultant from psychopathology is a peripheral issue, that it arises from society and the beliefs that people hold which are largely influenced by media and film (Curtis & Kelley, 2020a). Stigma about psychopathology, specifically pathological lying, can be addressed by exercising sociopolitical responsibilities through educating students, practitioners, and the general public (Blashfield & Burgess, 2007; Curtis & Hart, 2020a).

A decision not to recognize or provide a label for pathological lying can also pose problems. There is a robust history of clinical cases documenting people who suffer from pathological lying. As it stands, the failure to formally recognize these individuals prohibits a diagnosis and treatment (Curtis & Hart, 2020a). In fact, people who have been identified as pathological liars tend to receive other diagnoses, due to pathological lying not being recognized as a diagnostic entity (Curtis & Hart, 2020a). Thus, recognition of pathological lying as a diagnostic entity would promote scientific endeavors and provide clinicians with the tools to more fully help those who have historically been misdiagnosed, have not received treatment, or have not had effective treatments.

PATHOLOGICAL LYING: HISTORY AND NOMENCLATURE

More than a century of work on pathological lying has remained tucked away in case studies, mentioned in some neuroscience articles, alluded to within assessments, referenced within popular culture, and briefly mentioned in book chapters and encyclopedias. One of the great challenges in understanding pathological lying has been the fragmented state of the research and literature; there has not been an effort to consolidate and unify the important yet fragmented works. One conspicuous area of fragmentation around pathological lying is with nomenclature. Pathological lying has been referenced as pseudomania, pseudologia fantastica, mythomania, morbid lying, compulsive lying, and habitual lying. Dike and colleagues (2005) stated: "Pathological lying, *pseudologia fantastica*, mythomania and morbid lying are generally used interchangeably, although it remains debatable whether they all describe the same phenomenon" (p. 343).

One earlier term used was *pseudomania*. The root of pseudomania would be *pseudo* meaning fake, false, or lying, and mania meaning an excess. For example, in 1868 Wharton referred to a morbid lying propensity as pseudomania. The word was used within a legal context and referenced to as a psychiatric condition. In 1876, Peters used the word "pseudomania" to refer to a man who had an abhorrence of the truth so much that it was understood to be a disease. In psychology the word pseudomania was used by American psychologist G. Stanley Hall in 1890.

Hall (1890) used the term when discussing "pathological lies" that were less commonly found within children (p. 67). Hall stated that

> *pseudomania* supervenes where lies for others, and even self-deception, is an appetite indulged directly against every motive of prudence and interest. As man cannot be false to others if true to self, so he cannot experience the dangerous exhilaration of deceiving others without being in a measure his own victim, left to believe his own lie. Those who have failed in many legitimate endeavors learn that they can make themselves of much account in the world by adroit lying. These cases demand the most prompt and drastic treatment. (p. 68)

Aside from Hall's briefly using the term pseudomania and its sparse occurrences within legal contexts or debates of others, it did not gain much traction and largely did not become commonly used to refer to pathological lying. In some contemporary psychiatric contexts, the use of the term pseudomania does not refer to pathological lying but is used to refer to a false-positive diagnosis of mania, in which mania is typically associated with bipolar disorder (Braun et al., 1999; Swartz, 2003). Within the *Dictionary of Psychopathology* (Kellerman, 2009), *pseudomania* has been referenced as

> shame psychosis and equivalent to an enosiophobia. Here the person is fraught with apprehension about having possibly committed a crime. With some such individuals, even writing something in black and white can be an enormous challenge the person will refuse because of the fear that writing anything will turn out to be the confession of a crime. (p. 193)

Conversely, the term pseudomania can still be found listed within medical terminology and references. The term has fallen out of use in describing pathological lying and is now used to describe other conditions (e.g., Mosby, 2017).

Around the time Hall (1890) published on pathological lies and pseudomania, Anton Delbrück (1891), a German psychiatrist, published his work on pathological lying. Delbrück used the term *pseudologia phantastica* to refer to lying that was so far outside the parameters of normality that it was a pathological condition. Both pseudologia phantastica or pseudo-logia fantastica have been used, depending on the language and usage. Pseudologia fantastica can roughly be translated to false words of an extraordinary degree. According to Healy and Healy (1915), Delbrück coined the term pseudologia phantastica based on his work with five patients over several years. Delbrück believed these cases (which are discussed in Chapter 4) deserved a new and separate name that could describe the abnormal lying that was not accounted for by delusion or false memory. The term pseudologia phantastica was then adopted and used by other authors who followed Delbrück (Healy & Healy, 1915).

Pseudologia fantastica is a bit more descriptive than pseudomania because it more directly emphasizes a false word, or lie. Fantastica highlights the pathological aspect of a false word, in that the false words are of an extraordinary magnitude or size. Pseudologia fantastica is a term that can still be found in wide usage today. For example, the *Dictionary of Psychopathology* defines it as a

> symptom of Munchausen syndrome that can also be seen in psychopathic individuals who create stories because of a need for continuous external stimulation. It is thought that the person experiences the self as having an impoverished inner life, thereby requiring the creation of such endless external stimulations. Thus it is a fear of silence in the inner life and can also be seen in organically damaged individuals. (Kellerman, 2009, p. 193)

The American Psychological Association (APA; 2020a) *Dictionary of Psychology* defines *pseudologia fantastica* as

> a clinical syndrome characterized by elaborate fabrications, which are usually concocted to impress others, to get out of an awkward situation, or to give the individual an ego boost. Unlike the fictions of confabulation, these fantasies are believed only momentarily and are dropped as soon as they are contradicted by evidence. Typical examples are the tall tales told by people with antisocial personality disorder, although the syndrome is also found among malingerers and individuals with factitious disorders, neuroses, and psychoses. (para. 1)

In 1905, French psychiatrist Ernest Dupré used the word *mythomania* to refer to the pathological tendency to lie. The root of myth or mythos (μῦθος) means stories or falsehoods and mania meaning excessive, resulting in mythomania meaning to tell excessive falsehoods or untrue stories. Dupré indicated that the pathological tendency to lie was voluntary and conscious. He wrote that "pathological mythomania is constituted, in abnormal children as in adults, by the excess of duration and intensity, and finally by the abnormal nature of the mythopathic manifestations" (Dupré, para. 35). Dupré argued that pathological mythomania may be evidenced early in child development, where most children tell stories, fabricate details, simulate, or outright lie as a part of normal development. He suggested that in abnormal cases, instead of manifesting itself, in fact, as in the normal child, like a kind of imaginative sport and in the innocent form of the spontaneous play of exuberant psychic energies, mythical activity is put at the service, in abnormal subjects, of vicious tendencies, instinctive perversions or morbid appetites; it thus manifests itself as a particular mode of intellectual activity, directed by pathological feelings and therefore no longer represents an instrument of play, but a weapon of war, all the more dangerous the more intelligent the patient is (Dupré, 1905, para. 36).

Around the same time, in 1902, Emil Kraepelin, one of the founders of modern scientific psychiatry, published *Clinical Psychiatry: A Textbook for Students and Physicians* (Kraepelin, 1902/1912). Within his textbook, he discussed pathological lying and termed one who does so as the "morbid liar and swindler" in reference to Delbruck's pseudologia phantastica. He described four psychopathic personalities: born criminals, the unstable, the morbid liar and swindler, and pseudoquerulants (Kraepelin, 1902/1912). He indicated that the morbid liar exhibited a disorder that consisted of "a morbid hyperactivity of the imagination, inaccuracy of memory, and a certain instability of the emotions and volitions" (Kraepelin, 1902/1912, p. 526). Further, he suggested that one of the characteristic features of morbid lying was "the satisfaction which the patients derive from the willful falsifications of memory—the 'joy of lying'" (Kraepelin, 1902/1912, p. 527).

In the early 1900s, a variety of prominent scholars began to discuss pathological lying. Karl Jaspers (1913/1963) discussed pathological lying in his book titled *Allgemeine Psychopathologie* (*General Psychopathology*). He indicated that pathological lying was a group of falsifications that are not the result of false memory. Jaspers described pathological lying as "stories about the past which are pure fantasy are eventually believed by their inventor himself. Such falsifications range from harmless tall stories to a complete falsification of the whole past" (p. 77). He also indicated that pathological lying may be a manifestation found within children who have nervous disorders.

In 1915, Healy and Healy discussed the term pathological lying, more specifically as a psychological disorder. The Healys provided a definition of pathological lying, stating that it is

> falsification entirely disproportionate to any discernible end in view, engaged in by a person who, at the time of observation, cannot definitely be declared insane, feebleminded, or epileptic. Such lying rarely, if ever, centers about a single event; although exhibited in very occasional cases for a short time, it manifests itself most frequently by far over a period of years, or even a lifetime. It represents a trait rather than an episode. Extensive, very complicated fabrications may be evolved. This has led to the synonyms mythomania; pseudologia phantastica. (p. 1)

The definition paints a picture of pathological lying as excessive lying across situations by a person who does not exhibit other psychopathology or does not lie as a result of other psychological disorders or physiological conditions. Further, pathological lying is defined as a smaller portion of the population that has been engaged in excessive lying for a long duration. Healy and Healy (1915) also indicated that pathological lying was a trait rather than episodic. Lastly, it was suggested that the features of pathological lying have led to the synonyms of mythomania and pseudologia phantastica. Healy and Healy (1915) believed that these synonyms were different names for the same disorder. This position is also shared by the APA (2020a), as in its definitions of pseudologia phantastica and mythomania, the *APA Dictionary of Psychology* indicates "See also pathological lying."

Although many people reference the definition of pathological lying proposed by Healy and Healy (1915), the only consensus tends to be that there is "no consensus definition for pathological lying" (Dike et al., 2005). In 2005, Dike and colleagues revisited the concept of pathological lying and put forth a modified definition from Healy and Healy's (1915) original. They suggested a modification that was simplified and did not contain etiology. Dike and colleagues defined pathological lying as "a falsification entirely disproportionate to any discernible end in view, may be extensive and very complicated, and may manifest over a period of years or even a lifetime" (p. 343).

Other iterations of pathological lying have been used to convey the same phenomenon. For example, pathological lying may be called compulsive lying or habitual lying. Compulsive lying is documented by Dupré (1905) referencing compulsive lying vanity. Ford (1996), in his book on deceit, defined *pathological lying* as "lying that is compulsive or impulsive, occurs on a regular basis, and either does not seem to serve overt material needs of the person or has a self-defeating quality to it" (p. 133). Ford (1996) suggested that pathological lying was compulsive and suggested that compulsive liars have a low self-esteem. Dike (2020) recently alluded to the aspect of compulsive being paired with lying may be the influence of the American Psychiatric Association (1987) with descriptions of factitious disorder consisting of a compulsive feature.

Similarly, pathological lying has been referenced as habitual lying, historically and currently in popular culture. Essentially, habitual lying is descriptive, in that it captures the aspects of pervasiveness and chronicity, indicating, like Healy and Healy (1915), that it is not episodic or situational. Jaspers (1913/1963) used the term *habitual lying* when he discussed dementia due to organic cerebral processes. Ford (1996) discussed habitual lying as a type of pathological lying. Ford suggested that habitual liars lie for many reasons and tend to harm the lives of family, friends, and coworkers as well as make their own life difficult. Buzar and colleagues (2010) published a paper on habitual lying within a philosophy journal. The authors constructed an argument, putting forth criteria of lying and habitual lying, detailing the distinctions. They suggested that habitual lying is different from lying because it occurs in daily life, across professions, occurs more frequently, and is lying with intention in action (Buzar et al., 2010).

Treanor (2012) explored definitional constructions of pathological lying. She agreed with Dike and colleagues (2005) that there was not a consensus with regard to defining pathological lying. Treanor reported finding 32 total definitions of pathological lying within the literature; however, 17 of these definitions were original definitions. Subsequently, Treanor coded definitional themes, assigned the theme a score, and then combined the themes of past definitions into a synthesized definition of pathological lying. The result of coding themes led Treanor to propose a definition of pathological lying as

> the habitual, extensive and repeated production of falsifications often of a complicated and fantastic nature, which are entirely disproportionate to any discernible end in view. Often the lies can be easily verified as untrue and the possibility that the untruth may at any moment be demolished does nothing to abash the liar. Such lying is not determined by situational or external factors, the pseudologues' falsehoods are not told for personal procurement—profit and material reward or social advantage—do not govern the pseudologue's motivation to lie. Instead unconscious internalised motivations, such as self-esteem enhancement, defence, narcissistic gratification, and wish fulfilment predominate. When an external reason for lying is suspected the nature of the lies told are often far in excess of the parameters of that reason. The pseudologue can be held hostage to their lies and cease to be master over them. The pseudologue demonstrates an impaired ability to distinguish between fiction and reality and may partially convince him or herself that their fabrications have some basis in fact. The lying behaviours manifest over a period of years or even a lifetime and the onset can be traced back at least to adolescence or early adulthood. The pseudologue cannot be declared insane, feebleminded or epileptic and the lying cannot be accounted

for by an intellectual defect, illness, organic memory impairment or delusion. (pp. 65–66)

Although Treanor's (2012) definition is an interesting and informative summary of past definitions of pathological lying, it is likely too tangential and unwieldy to be useful in application.

PATHOLOGICAL LYING: A DEFINITION BASED ON THEORY AND RESEARCH

Although there has been a robust historical recognition of pathological lying, two enduring stumbling blocks have been disagreements about nomenclature and the absence of a widely agreed-on definition that can be used within research and practice. Regarding nomenclature, the use of multiple names for pathological lying has likely contributed to fragmentation and maybe even hinderance of the understanding and scientific study of the phenomenon. Arguably, before a definition can be advanced, basic nomenclature should be established. One of the six basic goals of any classification system is nomenclature (Blashfield & Burgess, 2007). The early work of Karl Jaspers (1913/1963) in setting a foundation for general psychopathology and Emil Kraepelin (1919) in establishing broad nomenclature for two classification categories represent the importance of terminology. Common nomenclature and diagnostic categories are essential for mental health professionals to communicate with each other and provide the basic building blocks by which clusters of symptoms are described and understood (Blashfield & Burgess, 2007).

There is a twofold dilemma regarding the nomenclature of pathological lying. On one hand, different terminology to explain and describe pathological lying existed before and during the establishment classification systems. It is evident that the lack of unifying language has led to disjointed work or even replication under a different name. While Jaspers (1913/1963) was certainly instrumental in compiling a survey of general psychopathology and a comprehensive text of a variety of psychopathologies, it was not designed as a formal classification tool. The first international classification, the "International List of Causes of Death," was implemented in 1893, primarily as a system that focused mostly on diseases that resulted in death (World Health Organization [WHO], 2021a, 2021b, 2021c). A plethora of terminology to refer to pathological lying proceeded the first edition of the *Diagnostic and Statistical Manual of Mental Disorders* (American Psychiatric Association, 1952). On the other hand, there has yet to be an authority (i.e., classification system or specific workforce committee) to provide or even adopt a framework for pathological lying. Cleary, several prominent individuals laid foundations for the recognition of pathological lying as a diagnostic entity. Hall (1890) put forth the existence of pathological lying within children, Healy and Healy (1915) laid out a compelling document for the existence of the disorder, and even Jaspers (1913/1963) documented pathological lying and pseudologia phantastica in his book on general psychopathology. Even so, pathological lying has yet to be recognized within major nosological classification systems, such as the fifth edition of the *Diagnostic and Statistical Manual of Mental Disorders* (*DSM-5*; American Psychiatric Association, 2013) and the *International Classification of Diseases, Eleventh Revision* (*ICD-11*; WHO, 2019). If classifications had recognized pathological lying, then the nomenclature would likely have crystallized into a common framework.

After establishing nomenclature, definitions help advance other goals of classification systems (Blashfield & Burgess, 2007). As indicated previously, definitions are important in the understanding of a construct and progressing scientific inquiry as well as achieving other goals of classification systems (e.g., prediction; Blashfield & Burgess, 2007). Therefore, we hope to advance understanding by suggesting the term pathological lying as the nomenclature for understanding the phenomenon referred to in the past and present as pseudomania, pseudologia fantastica, mythomania, compulsive lying, and habitual lying. The use of the term pathological lying appears to be endorsed by the large majority of scholars studying pathological lying (Treanor, 2012).

The various terms and definitions that have been proposed have certainly shed light on pathological lying and provided insight into commonalities. Treanor (2012) suggested that "while definitions identified throughout the literature, such as Healy and Healy's (1915), hold good face validity and make intuitive sense, their legitimacy is undermined by poor empirical and/or theoretical justification" (p. 65). Recently, we proposed a theoretical framework for understanding pathological lying (Curtis & Hart, 2020). This framework was based on a model to understand psychopathology (Curtis & Kelley, 2016, 2020a), the biopsychosocial model of psychopathology (Engel, 1996), and an alignment with the major nosological classification systems (i.e., *DSM-5* and *ICD-11*).

Drawing from the framework of previous definitions and case studies, grounded in the theory of psychopathology, and adhering to major nosological classification systems, we proposed a definition of pathological lying (Curtis & Hart, 2020b). Our definition was empirically tested and corroborated by our findings. We expand on the theory and research in subsequent chapters and discuss its utility for clinicians and researchers. Our work and theory led to the proposed definition of pathological lying as

> a persistent, pervasive, and often compulsive pattern of excessive lying behavior leading to clinically significant impairment of functioning in social, occupational, or other areas, causing marked distress, and posing a risk to the self or others, occurring for longer than a six month period. (Curtis & Hart, 2020b, p. 63)

RECONSIDERING THE PATHOLOGICAL LIAR

Bok (1999) argued that pathological liars are relatively harmless by asking one to consider "a pathological liar, known to all, and quite harmless; someone, perhaps, who is falsely immodest about athletic feats in his youth" (p. 126). This description flies in the face of the opening of this book, in that people tend to think of pathological liars as cold, calculated, manipulators. We would kindly disagree with Bok (1999) and assert that pathological lying is certainly not harmless, as our definition and research indicate. Our findings indicate that pathological lying carries a heavy toll, damaging relationships, causing dysfunction in many domains of life, and ultimately leaving a wake of distress (Curtis & Hart, 2020b).

We do not hold the position that pathological liars lack normal emotions and empathy or are out to wreak havoc at every opportunity. Although there are people who do lie with great frequency and may have malicious intentions, this does not broadly represent the overall group of people who engage in pathological lying. The stereotypical view that pathological liars are sinister could better be attributed to psychopathy. In the opening of Robert Hare's (1999) book *Without Conscience: The Disturbing World of the Psychopaths Among Us, psychopaths* are described as "social predators who charm, manipulate, and ruthlessly plow their way through life, leaving a broad trail of broken hearts, shattered expectations, and empty wallets" (p. xi). Pathological lying is sometimes conflated with psychopathy or antisocial personality disorder due to deceit being a symptom of those disorders (American Psychiatric Association, 2013; Hare, 1991). As Hare (1996) differentiated psychopathy from antisocial personality disorder, we too make a case that pathological lying is distinct from both of these psychopathologies.

For well over a century, pathological lying has been given many names and has been characterized in many ways. The study, diagnosis, and treatment of this intriguing phenomenon have been unfocused and faltering. We have written this book as a functional and cohesive source for clinicians and researchers to better understand pathological lying. We aim to demonstrate that previous accounts of various forms of disordered lying can be understood as a singular phenomenon. We also make the case that there is a common set of features among pathological liars. We hope that a unified terminology and definition around pathological lying might guide researchers and practitioners by offering a succinct, theory-driven, and empirically corroborated account of this disorder, which will serve as a guide for future research and as a reference for practitioners.

2

Normative Aspects of Lying

WHAT IS LYING?

A discussion of the patterns of lying in human cultures should begin with a delimitation and characterization of what is meant by the term. *Lying* has been defined numerous ways, but most definitions have as their core criterion that a person says something that is untrue. Obviously, however, not all untrue statements are lies. If someone says that California is the westernmost state (because they forgot about Hawaii), you would say that they are mistaken or that they are ignorant, not that they are a liar. As we dig deeper into the concept of lying, one can imagine instances where a person might be labeled a liar, even though what they said was actually true. A colleague recently asked if he was a liar and then recounted an interaction with his children. It was summer break, so all of the kids were home with him as he was trying to get some work done. The kids begged him to take them to the park to play. Having no interest in taking them to the park, he said, "We can't go today because it is supposed to rain."

https://doi.org/10.1037/0000305-002
Pathological Lying: Theory, Research, and Practice, by D. A. Curtis and C. L. Hart

He fully believed that rain was not in the forecast and that it would remain a sunny day with no precipitation. The children wandered off to find some other activity to occupy their time. A short time later, he heard his kids yelling that it was starting to rain. He glanced out the window and was surprised to see a downpour. Had he lied to his kids? As it turned out, he had not uttered an untruth. He said it would rain, and it did.

Consider further that people can easily deceive others by saying technically truthful things. If someone stated that a coworker lies a lot, it would likely leave the impression that the coworker is deeply deceptive. However, this crafty use of language truthfully means that the coworker lies on their bed every night. Technically truthful statements can be uttered in such a way that they successfully allow the deception of unwitting people. There are many other ways to create deceptively false impressions that do not require false statements to be uttered, such as with tone, body language, and context.

Most definitions of lying highlight intent as a key criterion. In the previous example of the man lying to his kids about rain, the actual accuracy of his statement was not particularly important in a person's judgment about his honesty. Many would say that he had lied because his intention was for his statement to deceive. The intent seems central to most people's concept of wrongdoings such as lying (Schein & Gray, 2018). Placing intent at the forefront, a common dictionary (*Merriam-Webster*) describes *lying* as "to make an untrue statement with *intent* to deceive." Deception researchers have also keyed in on intent in their definitions, describing a lie, for example, as "a message knowingly transmitted by a sender to foster a false belief or conclusion by the receiver" (Buller & Burgoon, 1996, p. 205).

Another point to consider is that spoken or written words need not be essential to a definition of lying. After all, there are many signs and signals that humans use to convey information to one another, including emojis, smoke signals, and silence. David Livingston Smith (2004) defined *lying* as "any form of behavior, the function of which is to provide others with false information or to deprive them of true information" (p. 14). He went on to say that breast implants are also lies and dispensed with any requirement for intention, whereas we prefer to constrain lying to the sphere of intentional communication. We agree with a definition provided by deception researcher Paul Ekman (1985) that lies require intention: "one person *intends* to mislead another, doing so deliberately, without prior notification of this purpose, and without having been explicitly asked to do so by the target" (p. 14). However, we part ways with Ekman because his definition allows for deceptive practices such as camouflage to be considered lies. Essentially, he argues that all deception is a lie, a position with which we disagree.

Another deception scientist, Aldert Vrij (2000), crafted a definition much like Ekman's, suggesting a *lie* is "a successful or unsuccessful deliberate attempt, without forewarning, to create in another a belief which the communicator considers to be untrue" (p. 6). Like Ekman, though, Vrij allows for any deception to be considered a lie. These are but a few examples of ways that scholars have defined lying. For a more complete review, see Mahon (2008).

We consider lying to be composed of three key elements. The liar must manipulate language, usually with words but sometimes with gestures or other signals that are reliably used to convey precise information to others. Second, the liar must believe the communication to convey an untrue representation of reality. Finally, the liar must intend to mislead another. On the basis of these criteria, and borrowing from Vrij and others, we define *lying* as "a successful or unsuccessful deliberate manipulation of language, without forewarning, to create in another a belief which the communicator considers to be untrue" (Hart, 2019).

WHY PEOPLE LIE

Many philosophers have examined and written about lying and deception, several expressing cautions or prohibitions against their use (e.g., Aquinas, 1947; Aristotle, 1941b; Kant, 1797/1996). People sometimes reason that lying is a necessity, arguing that they had no other choice but to lie. Some scholars who strongly advocate for strict adherence to truthfulness (e.g., Bok, 1978; Harris, 2013) concede that as morally reprehensible as lying might be, certain conditions render lying a necessity. For instance, people may condone lying to help spare an innocent life, where only by lying could one intervene to prevent a murder. The classic ethical thought experiment, often used as an objection to Kant's categorical imperative, illustrates a situation in which people may pardon a lie. The thought experiment asks you to consider that the Nazis came to your door looking for a person of Jewish faith who was hiding in your shed. Would you tell the truth? Even when people are not hand-wringing over decisions to spare another's life with being dishonest, people find plenty of reasons to lie or to justify their lying. Bok (1978) quipped, "The fact is that reasons to lie occur to most people quite often" (p. xvii). On the other hand, as Bok also noted, when there is not a reason or incentive to lie, people are almost universally honest, save for the rare person whose psychopathology drives them to lie without reason. Bok referred to this tendency toward honesty as the *principle of veracity*. Her argument was that there is a moral asymmetry between truth and lies. In the abstract, the truth imposes no moral cost because it is a mere description of reality. On the other hand, the lie is more weighty because it imposes on others a deprivation of their freedom to respond to the world as it actually is. Thus, Bok argued, the truth is the natural default position. There is not only a moral cost associated with lying; there is a cognitive one too. There is clear research evidence that lying is more cognitively demanding than telling the truth (Vrij et al., 2011). Additionally, a comprehensive meta-analysis shows that the work associated with generating a lie takes more time than telling the truth (Suchotzki et al., 2017). Thus, the cognitive burden of lying also leaves the truth as the default position, all else being equal. However, all else is often not equal. Sure, if the outcome of lying or telling the truth are equivalent, we will tell the truth. Why bother with the more effortful lie? But in many cases, no such equivalency exists. There are costs and benefits of telling the truth or lying, and in some cases, the cost of the truth is too high, so we lie.

Researchers have demonstrated what common sense tells each of us—incentives drive people to lie (Gneezy, 2005). When there is some advantage to be gained or some punishment to be avoided by shading the truth, people often choose dishonesty. For instance, in one study, researchers created a situation in which they incentivized lying or truth-telling (Bond et al., 2013). Half of the participants were incentivized to lie with the threat of a punishment. If they were truthful, they would be required to perform a boring task (watching a clock for 15 minutes), where if they lied, they would avoid the punishment. The results showed that incentives perfectly predicted who would lie and who would tell the truth. Those incentivized to lie all lied, and those not incentivized to lie all told the truth. In another set of studies, Levine et al. (2010) cleverly showed that when telling the truth is easy and there is no discernible benefit to lying, people are truthful. On the other hand, if the truth becomes an obstacle to achieving their goals, people seek other strategies, and lying is often a useful one. As Levine saw it, the truth and lies are both used for the same thing: achieving goals. If goals can economically be snared with honesty, people go with that default, because after all, the truth is the easiest to produce. Across three studies, Levine showed that when there was no incentive to lie, people chose to respond honestly almost 100% of the time. However, when he incentivized lying across a number of scenarios (e.g., cheating for extra prize money in a trivia game), people lied more than 60% of the time. As predicted, if the lie makes achieving a goal easier than the truth would, people resort to lying. Of course, people do not just consider the ease of lying or telling the truth in the moment. There is a consideration of future consequences. If I lie to you today to achieve my goal and you find out, you may make it harder for me to achieve my next goal tomorrow. You may also tell people that I am a liar, sullying my reputation. When telling lies, one must consider the vast calculus of immediate and future costs and rewards across expansive, interrelated social networks. The consequences of the truth or the lie right now can ripple out to distant shores.

Beyond broad theories of why people lie, the specific motivations that drive people to lie in their day-to-day lives can be examined.

MOTIVATIONS FOR LYING

Paul Ekman (2021), who has been studying deception for decades, reported that across his many studies, people tended to lie for only a handful of reasons. These included lying to avoid punishment, to secure rewards, to shield others from punishment, to shield oneself from physical harm, to enhance oneself in the eyes of others, to extricate oneself from socially awkward situations, to escape potential embarrassment, to maintain one's privacy, and to control others behavior by manipulating the information they have access to. DePaulo et al. (1996) also examined the reasons people give for lying. They found that most people did not appear to lie to malevolently manipulate others or for some immediate financial gain. Rather, most seemed to lie for more vulnerable psychological reasons. Many of the lies they told were with the goal of avoiding criticism, embarrassment, or disapproval. Lippard (1988) also explored the motivations behind lying and deception. She identified eight motivations for telling lies. The most common reason was conflict avoidance, followed by protecting others, self-protection, securing or holding resources, excuses, increasing or decreasing affiliation with others, manipulating others, lying for the benefit of a third party, and joking. Drouin and colleagues (2016) asked people about their motivation for lying online. The majority of responses fell into two categories. The first was a motivation to gain more acceptance or attention by presenting oneself in a more flattering light. For instance, people presented themselves as being more attractive, interesting, or adventurous than they actually were. The other common motivation was privacy and safety. For instance, people would conceal or lie about their location, identity, or age to avoid exploitation.

Much of the deception research has been conducted in WEIRD locations (i.e., Westernized, educated, industrialized, rich, democratic), and much of that has been conducted in the United States and a handful of European countries. Thus, it has been difficult to determine whether the motivations to lie that have been found in much of the research represent some human universals or just the peculiarities of the locations in which the data were collected. Recently, a team of researchers cast a wider net collecting data on motivations to lie not just from the United States but from a variety of countries including historically understudied locales such as Guatemala, Egypt, Saudi Arabia, and Pakistan (Levine et al., 2016). They found that there was surprising similarity in motivations across countries, although there were some small idiosyncratic variations. Combined, the motivations were as follows, from most common to least:

concealing personal transgressions: 21.5%
creating an economic advantage: 15.6%

creating a nonmonetary gain or advantage: 14.7%

creating an excuse to avoid someone: 14.4%

creating a favorable impression of oneself: 7.8%

helping others: 5.1%

for humor or for a joke: 5.1%

to harm someone else: 4.2%

being sociable and polite: 2.4%

no apparent motive or goal: 1.5%

The remaining 16% could not recall a lie, indicated a lie that did not fit into the above categories, or provided insufficient data for coding. So, we can see that people lie when there is an incentive, and there tends to be a common group of incentives that motivate people's lies.

Deception researchers have also discussed motivations to lie as encompassing a variety of dimensions. Vrij (2008) discussed three dimensions of motivations to lie: (a) the person who benefits (self vs. others), (b) lying for gain or to avoid loss, and (c) lying for materialistic or for psychological reasons. Thus, some deception literature may discuss motivations to lie based on the category of locus of benefit, whereas others may discuss motivations to lie based on a behavioral perspective, examining the consequences of telling previous lies. Elsewhere we have proposed and discussed a model to understand and separate motivations of lying (see Hart & Curtis, in press). When studying deception, the various motivations to lie are not different from the motivations to tell the truth (Levine et al., 2010). That is, both lies and truths are told to achieve some end through communication.

WHY PEOPLE ARE HONEST

When exploring questions of why people lie, it is equally worthwhile to ask why people do not lie more than they do. By most people's reports, the vast majority of their lies go undetected (Vrij, 2000). If people can consistently twist the truth without anyone realizing it, why not do it regularly? Why does honesty seem to be a central feature of our nature? Our data show us that most people are honest most of the time. People could easily lie, yet they opt not to. And even if they are dishonest, they don't always lie to their maximal advantage (Mazar et al., 2008). They tell small lies rather than bigger, more self-serving ones. There are a few theories about what constrains lying. Dan Ariely (2012) argued that people attempt to remain largely honest so that they can maintain the ability to view themselves as honest—and ultimately good—people. He cited numerous examples in his own research where people could lie to claim a large payout but instead told a lesser lie and received a smaller payout. He argued that people have a deep-seated need to maintain a self-concept in which they can see themselves in a positive light, referred to as *self-concept maintenance* (Ariely, 2012; Mazar et al., 2008). By only being a little dishonest, people can continue to view themselves as essentially good people. In effect, people are honest so that they can look at themselves in the mirror each day without feeling guilt and shame. Lying can be a behavior that challenges one's own perception of being an honest person, leading to cognitive dissonance— the discrepancy between behavior and perceptions of self-consistency (Festinger, 1957).

Ironically, a word of caution is warranted when discussing the aforementioned work of Dan Ariely. Recently, some of his work has been retracted from journals because of clear indications of fraud. Additionally, others have suggested that he has made claims about studies that he, in fact, had not actually carried out (O'Grady, 2021). Although we won't impugn his entire body of scholarly work here, we do believe that some caution is warranted in accepting his findings.

Another theory about pervasive honesty can be examined through a Darwinian lens. The argument starts with the observation that people are largely honest, and then works backward. We can see that most human communications are truthful ones. This is consistent across cultures. From an evolutionary perspective, this surely means that honesty is, or at least was, adaptive in human evolution history. That is, it seems that humans who were largely honest tended to survive and reproduce at higher rates than those who were not. On the other hand, given that deception seems to offer obvious self-serving advantages yet is not widespread, it suggests that, over evolutionary time, lying must have carried considerable costs.

The evolutionary psychology framework suggests that to understand human honesty, one must first understand that humans evolved as a highly social species. We can examine humans in hunter–gatherer societies, living much as our ancestors did for hundreds of thousands of years. Anthropologists' studies of hunter–gatherer societies find that they are highly cooperative and are highly dependent on each other. That intense cooperation is not just a matter of politeness; it is a matter of survival (Laland, 2017; Pennisi, 2009). In hunter–gatherers, such as the Hadza of Tanzania, sharing food and resources through a connection of social networks and banding together in coalitional defense is the key to not meeting an early grave (Apicella et al., 2012). Life for our ancestors was hard. Food was not always plentiful, and danger from predators and other aggressive humans was always a possibility. By cooperating with food, people were able to share the bounty of others' resources when they might have otherwise starved (Lavi & Friesem, 2019). Likewise, they could count on rallying support from tribe members if enemies came into camp with homicidal intentions. Through cooperation, a bad day for any person was much less likely to result in death, as other group members aided each other in survival.

However, people do not cooperate randomly (Delton et al., 2011; Heintz et al., 2016; Mohtashemi & Mui, 2003). Rather, they tend to be choosy with the selection of cooperative partners. People cooperate with those who reciprocate, or at least those who seem like they will cooperate. They need not have a history of reciprocating with us. They can merely have a reputation as a good cooperative partner. People who lie and cheat instead of cooperating, referred to as free-riders, tend to be punished. In human terms, this punishment sometimes means being ostracized from the group. Being ostracized and forced to fend for oneself would have dramatically decreased the odds of surviving and reproducing. Those who were reliable cooperators lived to pass on copies of their genes. Those who consistently lied and cheated were rejected, and did not pass on their genes. The idea is that people work hard to cultivate and maintain reputations as people who can be trusted.

Humans go out of their way to signal that loyalty. People are especially keen to demonstrate honesty when their reputation is on the line

(Gneezy et al., 2018). Ironically, people sometimes lie just to prove that they are trustworthy. For instance, imagine someone offered to pay you to complete a task. Imagine you told them that it would take you between 60 and 90 hours to complete the task, and they agreed to pay you per hour. Now imagine that it took you exactly 90 hours to complete the task. In just this type of scenario, people tended to lie and underreport how long it took them to complete the task (Choshen-Hillel et al., 2020). That is, they actually lied and took a pay cut rather than reporting honestly and being paid the correct amount. The reason seemed to be that people worried they would be perceived as cheats and a liars if they claimed to have required exactly the full 90 hours. After all, claiming that the job took exactly 90 hours is what one would expect a real cheater would do. In another line of research, psychologists found that people attempt to prove that they are trustworthy and loyal to people by lying for those people (Levine & Schweitzer, 2015). For instance, a good way to demonstrate one's loyalty to a friend would be to lie for them to get them out of a pinch. Not surprisingly, those who are willing to tell lies for their team were actually perceived as being more trustworthy.

Behaviorism and learning theory would indicate that honesty is largely brought about through principles of conditioning and social learning (Bandura et al., 1961; Pavlov, 1960; Skinner, 1938). From this perspective, honesty has been reinforced socially and within relationships across the lifespan. Stories have been told throughout time that are intended to teach honesty. For example, stories like George Washington and the cherry tree or Aesop's fables are usually designed to promote honesty. In fact, research has found that stories that depicted positive consequences from being honest (e.g., George Washington) deterred lying behaviors more than stories that discussed the punishing consequences of lying (e.g., the boy who cried wolf; Lee et al., 2014). In addition to telling these moral stories, parents tend to strongly convey the value of honesty (Heyman et al., 2009). Honesty becomes associated with positive outcomes and is reinforced.

In the same vein, Levine and colleagues (2010) indicated that "it is only when the truth poses an obstacle to goal attainment, regardless of what that goal might be, that people entertain the possibility of being deceptive" (p. 273). Thus, people are generally honest and only lie when the truth is problematic (Levine et al., 2010). Honesty is the default position of most people, referred to as the truth-default theory (TDT; Levine, 2014b, 2020). Levine (2020) stated that "people lie for a reason but the motives behind truthful and deceptive communication are the same. While the truth is consistent with the person's goals, he or she will almost always communicate honesty" (p. 152). Levine (2020) argued that pathological lying may be a case where lies are told without a reason. However, one issue is the ability to discern what a person's reason may be or even if the individual is consciously aware of their reasons.

NORMATIVE LYING

In the clinical literature, most historical uses of the term *pathological lying* have treated it as a form or a symptom of a psychological disorder (Dike, 2008; Healy & Healy, 1915). Principally, it has been viewed as a psychiatric condition with frequent and pervasive lying as the core feature. In addition to its use as a clinical term, pathological liar has also been a term in the common vernacular for more than 100 years, along with similar terms such as *habitual liar* and *compulsive liar*. In the common parlance, these terms are used to refer not to a mental disorder but simply to a person who lies beyond acceptable norms. For instance, in 1718, Nicholas Clark wrote, "For the habitual liar is looked upon with scorn and contempt, and hardly believed when he speaketh Truth" (p. 193). The term habitual liar, in that sense, did not connote a mental illness. Rather, it suggested a moral defect.

Our research suggests that outside of the sphere of mental health professionals, people seem to treat pathological liar, compulsive liar, and habitual liar as synonyms, an observation first made by Healy and Healy (1915). In all cases, the general conception is that these are terms used to describe a person who lies excessively and far outside the bounds of normalcy. We have asked hundreds of laypeople if they have ever met or known a pathological liar (Hart, Beech, & Curtis, 2022). With the majority of people affirming that they have, it seems to be a fairly common experience. Yet when asked to describe the pathological liar, there was rarely any mention of mental illness, which supports our position that most using the term simply mean to label a person who lies a lot. This leads us to the obvious question of what amounts to a lot of lying. For that matter, what is a normal amount of lying?

NONACADEMIC SURVEYS

In 1991, two advertising executives, James Patterson and Peter Kim, conducted a massive study in which they anonymously interviewed thousands of Americans in a nationwide study. One of the topics they examined was lying. On the question of whether people viewed honesty as a moral imperative, they found that two thirds of Americans felt that there was nothing wrong with telling a lie. They also reported that 91% of the participants said that they lie regularly. The vast majority indicated that they lie to those closest to them, including friends, family, and spouses.

A 2021 survey carried out for the website Zety.com collected data via an online survey from 1,034 Americans about lies they tell to get out of work, such as falsely calling in sick. They found that 96% of respondents admitted to lying to get out of work. Most of them (91%) said their lies had never been detected (Tomaszewski, 2021). A 2004 survey conducted by *Reader's Digest* polled more than 2,500 people about various forms of dishonesty such as lying (Kalish, 2004). Of their respondents, 98.5% admitted to lying or some other form of dishonesty at some point. Thus, given the results from informal surveys, it seems that most Americans are less than completely honest.

One issue with measuring lying is that we must rely on self-report, and there are serious questions about the degree to which we can trust those reports. For instance, heterosexual men in the United States report using 1.6 billion condoms during their sexual escapades each year (Stephens-Davidowitz, 2017). However, market analysis shows that only 600 million condoms are sold in the country each year. Either reusing condoms has become fashionable or people's self-reports are inaccurate. Self-report inaccuracies can arise from a lack of awareness. Benjamin Franklin (1750) noted, "There are three things extremely hard: steel, a diamond, and to know one's self." For instance, people tend to touch their faces hundreds of times per day, but these numerous spontaneous self-touches largely occur without awareness (Harrigan et al., 1987; Kwok et al., 2015). Even when people are aware of their behavior, their ample capacity for forgetting limits their ability to correctly report on that behavior (Bartlett, 1932; Ebbinghaus, 1885). Finally, when people are asked to self-report, they may choose to respond inaccurately. That is, they lie (Brenner & DeLamater, 2016). Lying on self-report surveys is certainly more likely when the questions are about legally or morally prohibited behaviors. This raises the obvious question in assessing the frequency of lying. If people say that they rarely lie, might they simply be lying to us?

The truth is that researchers ultimately do not know with certainty that people honestly report about their lying. Researchers have identified a number of techniques that increase the rates of honest responding (Moshagen et al., 2010; Vésteinsdóttir et al., 2019). For instance, when asking questions about sensitive topics, allowing the participant to conceal their identity and remain anonymous reduces the likelihood of underreporting or overreporting behaviors out of embarrassment. One way that researchers have validated self-report measures is by first having participants fill out a self-report measure and afterward asking those same questions of the participants during a polygraph examination (J. P. Clark & Tifft, 1966; G. S. Green, 1990). Those types of studies generally show that people's self-reports align with what appears to be their truthful responses to the same questions while under polygraph examination.

There is some strong scientific evidence that self-report measures of lying are valid. In two studies (Halevy et al., 2014), researchers asked people to report how often they lie. Subsequently, the researcher had those same participants play a game. In the game, it was possible to lie and cheat to come out ahead and achieve greater rewards. The researchers were able to secretly record whether participants lied and cheated. Across both studies, they found that those people who lied and cheated the most were also the people who self-reported that they lie the most.

DIARY STUDIES

The first scientific examinations of lie frequency were carried out by the psychologist, DePaulo and her colleagues in the 1990s (DePaulo et al., 1996; Kashy & DePaulo, 1996). In those studies, the researchers recruited dozens of participants and then asked them to record every lie they told, big or small, in a personal diary for an entire week. In the two samples from DePaulo et al. (1996), college student participants reported telling an average of 1.96 (*SD* = 1.63) lies per day, and a somewhat older (mean age = 34) group of nonstudent adults who were recruited from continuing education programs at a community college told an average of 0.97 (*SD* = 0.98) lies per day. Over the full week, 95% of all participants reported telling a lie. Most of the lies were told fairly spontaneously, without much forethought or planning.

Diary studies are considered to be quite a good method for collecting accurate data, given that retrospective data collection relying on human memory is fraught with forgetfulness and memory distortions (D. R. Anderson et al., 1985). Nonetheless, diary methods still rely on participants accurately recognizing and recording events as they occur. Also, as the diary recording occurs after the event, even if only a short time after, errors in memory may still be a problem. Although some evaluations purport that diary methods are far superior to retrospective survey techniques (Conrath et al., 1983; Wind & Lerner, 1979), other findings (Schulz & Grunow, 2012) suggest that the two methods produce congruent results.

In somewhat of a replication of DePaulo's studies, Hancock et al. (2004), carried out a lie frequency study in which they had 28 participants keep a tally of every lie they told over 7 days. They found that their sample told an average of 1.58 (*SD* = 1.02) lies per day. In a variation of DePaulo's studies, Hancock et al. distinguished between lies told face-to-face versus those told via electronic communication. Their analysis showed that the per day average was 1.03 (*SD* = .68) for face-to-face lies, 0.35 (*SD* = .24) for lies told over the phone, 0.18 (*SD* = .20) for those told via instant messaging, and 0.06 (*SD* = .07) for lies told in email communications. Although they found that people told the most lies when communicating face-to-face, this seemed to be a consequence of the fact that most communications happen face-to-face rather than people necessarily being more dishonest via any one channel of communication. They did not collect data that would allow for valid conclusions to be drawn about the rates of deception via the various channels of communication.

In 2008, George and Robb offered yet another quasi-replication of DePaulo et al.'s (1996) original diary study. Their study consisted of two samples of college students, with 25 students in each sample. In both samples, they had participants record each time they lied for 7 days. They further broke down the format of communication into face-to-face communication and various phone and electronic media. In the first sample, participants reported lying 0.59 times per day. In the second sample, participants reported lying an average of 0.9 times per day. Most of the lies took place face-to-face or over the phone, but again, this seems to be a consequence of more communication taking place over those formats, and they offered no data that would allow valid conclusions to be drawn about relative rates of lying via the different formats.

SURVEY STUDIES

Another common way of estimating lie frequency is through scientific surveys. For instance, Grant et al. (2019) found that in a large sample of college students, 18% reported that they lied every single day. Drouin et al. (2016) surveyed 272 adults and found that 84% of U.S. adults said that they would lie to people online (i.e., social media, chat rooms, dating sites, and other websites). However, to gauge the frequency of lying, researchers must ask participants to recollect how many lies they told over the course of a specified span of time. The results largely mirror what has been found in diary studies. Serota et al. (2010) found that 92% of people reported lying during the past week and told an average of 1.65 ($SD = 4.45$) lies in the preceding 24 hours. In another sample, Serota and Levine (2015) found that people reported telling an average of 1.66 lies per day ($SD = 2.37$). In our own survey of 653 people (Hart, Beech, & Curtis, 2022), they reported telling an average of 1.4 lies per day. In another study, participants indicated that they had told an average of 1.61 lies in the past 24 hours (Verigin et al., 2019). There are still more survey studies, but most replicate this typical finding that people report lying, on average, about one to two times per day.

Although almost all people lie and seem to do so with some regularity, some people certainly seem to lie more than the rest. Serota and colleagues (2010) were the first to closely examine the distribution of lying within large samples. In their study titled "The Prevalence of Lying in America: Three Studies of Self-Reported Lies," they reanalyzed two data sets from previously published research reports on lying. While those previous studies had examined the rates of lying, Serota and colleagues wanted to understand how the data were spread out. For instance, if you are told that the average person tells two lies per day, there are a number of patterns that could give rise to that average. For instance, every person in the sample could lie exactly two times, yielding a mean of two, or most people could tell one lie with a smaller group telling 10 lies each, also yielding a mean of two. It is often informative to move beyond just looking at a single point estimate such as the mean and scrutinize the shape of the entire distribution. This is what Serota and colleagues did. What they found was that the distribution was extremely skewed. It turned out that when people reported how many times they lied in the past 24 hours, the average was around one or two. If one looks more closely at the distribution, though, one will see that most people report being fairly honest over a day, but a small minority does a large amount of lying. This small group of prolific liars inflated the mean, causing the average to provide a distorted depiction of how often a typical person lies.

Serota and colleagues (2010) went on to collect a large sample of their own. Their sample was a very representative national sample of 1,000 adults from various parts of the United States. They asked participants the following question:

> Think about where you were and what you were doing during the past 24 hours, from this time yesterday until right now. Listed below are the kinds of people you might have lied to and how you might have talked to them, either face-to-face or some other way such as in writing or by phone or over the Internet. In each of the boxes below, please write in the number of times you have lied in this type of

situation. If you have not told any lies of a particular type, write in "0."
In the past 24 hours, how many times have you lied? (p. 8)

Again, they found the same pattern where most people reported being particularly honest, and a small minority seemed to be doing most of the lying. When people reported how many lies they had told in the preceding 24 hours, the average was 1.65 lies ($SD = 4.45$). However, if one ranked the participants from highest to lowest, the person in the middle of that distribution (the median) reported telling zero lies. In fact, zero was the most common response (the mode). A full 60% of their participants reported telling no lies. Even among the remaining 40% that did report lying, most of them only told one or two. If so many people were saying they told no lies, why was the average almost two? This was a case of the average being inflated by a handful of people who were doing a whole lot of lying.

TIME-FRAME CONSIDERATIONS

When the data showed that on a given day, 60% of people told zero lies, it is tempting to conclude that most people were honest. However, it is important to recognize how lying was being measured in those studies. A critical decision in measuring lie frequency is selecting the ideal time frame. If we ask people how many times they have lied in the past year, for example, they are unlikely to have an accurate recall due to forgetting and due to the large number of instances that must be tabulated. On the other hand, if we ask them how many times they have lied in the past minute, we are unlikely to record any lies because most people are unlikely to be speaking in any given minute, let alone speaking deceptively. Ideally, we will select a frame of time that is both long enough for us to observe behavior occurring, but brief enough to avoid the problem of forgetfulness and the problem of trying to mentally tally a large number of instances. As an indication of the issue, consider that when Serota et al. (2010) asked people how many times they had lied over a single day, 60% reported having told no lies. That data point erroneously gives the impression that most people do not lie. We would see the same pattern if we asked people about any other relatively low-frequency behaviors, such as eating pizza, going to see a movie, or cutting one's fingernails. We do know that most people engage in these behaviors, but they just don't do so regularly enough for us to detect them by observing them on a single day. This is no trivial matter. The primary problem with asking people how many times they have lied in one day is that the majority will look identical—that is, they report zero. However, we know that the group is unlikely to actually be uniform. If we were to observe them over numerous days instead of just one, we would see that some who told zero lies over 1 day would still have told zero lies over 3 or 4 days. But some others who told zero lies over 1 day would surely tell one or more lies by Day 3 or 4. By restricting the range of observation to a single day, we are failing to capture differences between people that actually do exist. For this reason, we strongly advocate for avoiding solely measuring lies over a 1-day period.

Fortunately, researchers have measured lie frequency in longer time frames. DePaulo et al. (1996) recorded lies over a week; they found that 99% of their student sample and 91% of their community sample had told at least one lie. In both of George and Robb's (2008) two student samples, 96% lied over a week. Serota et al. (2010) found that 92% lied during the past week. Across two of our samples (Beech et al., 2021), 87% and 84% reported that they told at least one lie per week. In data from another of our studies (Hart, Beech, & Curtis, 2022), only 45% reported having told a lie over the past 24 hours, similar to what Serota and colleagues found when asking that question. However, 84% said they told at least one lie in a typical week. When one looks at lying on any given day, most people seem entirely honest. When one looks at lying over an entire week, the vast majority of people are liars.

Returning to the issue of skewed distributions in the frequency of lying, we would like to draw the focus back to the fact that some people lie a lot. This is an important point. Rather than simply concluding that the average person tells one to two lies per day, a much more accurate representation is that most people lie fairly infrequently, but a small proportion of people lie a lot. The bulk of the lying is being done by just a small minority. This is particularly important as we begin to discuss normal versus abnormal lying. If we wish to examine lying that is pathological, we focus our analysis on a small handful of people. For instance, Serota and colleagues (2010) found that just 5% of the people in their study accounted for half of the lies that were being told. One person in their study reported telling 53 lies in 1 day. Some do seem to lie abnormally.

ATTITUDES ABOUT NORMALITY

But what is a normal versus abnormal amount of lying? We carried out two studies in which we asked people what a normal or average amount of lying was (Hart, Beech, & Curtis, 2022). The first sample (Group 1) was 251 people recruited via Amazon Mechanical Turk. The average age was 37. The gender breakdown was 60% were men and 40% were women. In a second sample (Group 2), we recruited 387 people from the general population through social media and email solicitations. The average age was 33. The gender breakdown was 66% women, 31% men, and 1% indicated other. We first asked them how often they thought the average or typical person lies per week. Group 1 responded with an average of 13.31 lies (median and mode were both 5), which equates to 1.90 lies per day. Group 2 had an average of 9.83 (median and mode both equaled 5), which equates to 1.40 lies per day. So, across these two samples, it looks like people think that others are telling about one to two lies per day. It was surprising to see people's estimates of others actually align with the lie frequency reported in other studies.

We also wanted to know how people perceived abnormal lying. Specifically, we asked both groups of people how many lies someone would need to tell to be considered a habitual, compulsive, or pathological liar. Our first finding was that people seemed to treat those three terms as synonyms because the answers they gave were uniform across the terms. Across both samples, participants indicated that telling an average of nine lies per day would warrant labeling a liar as habitual, compulsive, or pathological (medians and modes were five). In sum, it looks like people report lying approximately one to two times per day, they think others also normally lie one to two times per day, and they think someone has a significantly abnormal level of lying if they tell nine or more lies per day (although the median of five might be a more reliable figure).

CONCLUSION

This chapter was about normative lying, so we have examined that lying which is typical or characteristic of the general populace. Our conclusions are that most people have lied, but lying is not necessarily frequent. Although lies are quite varied, people tend to lie for only a handful of core reasons, mainly to help or avoid harm for themselves or for others. People lie when the truth gets in the way of more important goals. Close to 100% of people report lying at some point in their lives. When we look at lying over a week, around 90% of people say they lie. When we examine lying over a single day, it looks like the average is one or two lies, although the majority report telling none and a few tell a lot. People estimate that their fellow citizens tell an average of one or two lies per day. On average, they see nine or more lies per day as a sign of a real problem. As we continue forward in this analysis of lying, we next examine what differentiates those who lie a little from those who lie a lot.

3

Characteristics of People Who Lie a Lot

PROLIFIC VERSUS NONPROLIFIC LIARS

Most people have probably known someone who was notably trustworthy and truthful. What these truthful individuals said could be counted on to be correct and genuine, having communicated sincerely, earnestly, and without obfuscation. Those people were honest. But to varying degrees, most people are not. Some people lie a little and some others lie a lot. For instance, in one of our studies (Hart et al., 2019), our participants reported telling an average of 2.39 lies in the preceding 24 hours, but one person reported telling 20 lies that day. In another of our studies (Hart, Beech, & Curtis, 2022), our participants reported telling an average of 13.18 lies per week (a little less than two per day), yet several people admitted telling more than 100 lies per week. In yet another study of ours, the total group reported telling an average of five lies per week, but several people reported telling at least 100. In fact, the top 10% of liars in that study told

https://doi.org/10.1037/0000305-003
Pathological Lying: Theory, Research, and Practice, by D. A. Curtis and C. L. Hart

52% of the lies (Hart, Curtis, & Randell, 2022). Other researchers have found similar patterns where a small number of people tell most of the lies (DePaulo et al., 1996; Halevy et al., 2014; Serota et al., 2010; Serota & Levine, 2015). In this chapter, we discuss characteristics of the big liars and how they are different from the rest of the population.

In 1896, Vilfredo Pareto, an Italian economist, published an idea that has subsequently become known as the *Pareto principle*. Pareto's idea was really more of an observation. He noticed that for any set of outcomes, the bulk of instances can be attributed to a relatively small proportion of causal agents. For instance, when it comes to income, the majority of income is generated by a proportionally small group of extremely high earners. When it comes to sales, the bulk of sales in a given company are produced by a relatively small proportion of salespeople. Pareto noticed this trend followed approximately an 80–20 split, where 80% of the outcomes are accounted for by 20% of the causes. For instance, most people probably spend 80% of their time on their smartphones using only 20% of the apps. The Pareto principle is a form of power law distribution. In statistics, power laws can describe patterns in which a small number of cases are clustered at one end of a distribution, accounting for a large proportion of the occurrences. For instance, there are a handful of billionaires who hold the majority of wealth in the United States. The rest of the populace, although varying in degree of wealth, hold much, much less. In the case of wealth, a small amount of wealth is the most common occurrence, while having extreme amounts of wealth is statistically rare. Serota and colleagues (2010) were the first to recognize that lying also follows a power law distribution, where most lies are told by a small proportion of the population. In their sample of 1,000 people, the participants reported telling a total of 1,646 lies in the preceding 24 hours; however just 5.3% of their sample told 50% of the lies. So, 53 people told an average of 16 lies each, where the remaining 947 people told an average of less than one lie each. This pattern of results has been replicated numerous times and seems to be a robust finding (DePaulo et al., 1996; Halevy et al., 2014; Hart et al., 2019; Serota & Levine, 2015).

The fact that lying seems to fit a power law function means that talking about the "average liar" is complicated. The distribution is so skewed that the average may offer a somewhat biased representation of the group. In our research, we are interested in studying the biggest liars—those who seem to lie considerably more than most people. Essentially, we are searching for very abnormal liars. So how do we find them? Well, the obvious approach would be to measure how much people lie and then simply select those who lie the most.

OUTLIERS

An outlier is a statistical anomaly. For instance, the average net worth of all American families is $746,820, and the median is $121,760 (Bhutta et al., 2020). However, in 2020, Jeff Bezos, the founder of Amazon, became the first person with a net worth of $200 billion (Ponciano, 2020). That is more than one and a half million times the median net worth in America. Jeff Bezos is an anomaly. If we hope to understand people who lie a lot, it is useful to study the outliers—those who lie much more than the typical person—the "outliars." But what constitutes an outlier in the context of lying? Is it someone who tells three lies a day? Four? Ten? How do we decide what the cutoff is? The identification of outliers is always arbitrary. Even if someone comes up with a mathematical rule for identifying outliers, the selection of that particular rule is arbitrary. There are numerous mathematical rules to aid data analysts in identifying the outlying cases. Some are well-suited for a normal distribution of data (e.g., Tukey, 1977), still other more advanced techniques have been developed to help identify the outliers in skewed distributions (e.g., Meropi et al., 2018). Recall that lying in a population seems to be substantially skewed, with most people lying very little and a small few lying a lot, so most standard techniques are of little use.

Ultimately, identifying outliers is a process in which the analyst subjectively is surprised by some distant data points and then, often, generates a subjectively chosen mathematical rule for separating the surprising values from the rest (Collett & Lewis, 1976). A visual inspection of the lying data does indeed reveal some surprising data points, with some people indicating that they are surprisingly honest and some reporting that they are shockingly deceptive. For instance, in some of our data, people have reported that they have not lied in more than a year, where the typical person indicates it has only been a day or two since their last lie (Hart, Curtis, & Randell, 2022). In that same data set, others reported lying dozens of times per day, while the typical person only lied once or twice.

People have a natural inclination to organize and understand their world through categorization, so some might seek to draw an arbitrary line to separate the typically honest people from the big liars. We have considered that issue. When we have visualized our data sets, we noticed that the top 5% of liars seem to account for a disproportionately large proportion of all of the lies being told. Interestingly, we found that Halevy et al. (2014) also identified the top 5% of liars as the "frequent liars" worthy of more attention—5% told 40% of the lies in their study. In one of our studies, for that top 5%, the median number of lies they told per week was 33 (Hart, Curtis, & Randell, 2022). For the remaining 95% of people, their median lies per week was two. In a second study, the top 5% told a median of 30 lies per week, and the rest told two (Hart, Beech, & Curtis, 2022). So, if we decide that the top 5% will be considered the big liars, we can see that the typical big liar tells about 15 to 17 times more lies than the rest of people, the typically honest.

Another way of separating out the big liars from the rest is to rely on people's opinions of what constitutes an abnormal amount of lying. As we noted in the previous chapter, we asked several hundred people how many lies someone would need to tell for them to be viewed as a problematic liar (Hart, Beech, & Curtis, 2022). The median response was five lies per day, which, coincidentally, is the median number of lies the top 5% report telling on a typical day. So, five lies per day or the top 5% of liars seems to be a reasonable rule of thumb for separating out the biggest liars from the rest.

There are other statistical means to examine lie frequency. Serota and Levine (2015) suggested a Poisson distribution, also referred to as a model of rare events, to identify prolific liars. Drawing from Cox and Lewis (1966), Serota and Levine (2015) suggested the use of an index of dispersion (D) to decide whether the data fit a distribution, where $D > 1$ is considered overdispersed, $D < 1$ (not 0) are likely normally distributed, and $D \approx 1$ as a fit of the Poisson distribution. They reported that when the sample data consisted of participants who told 0 to 4 lies, then a value of $D = 0.97$ was found. Thus, they determined that five lies or more was considered prolific lying.

Another similar statistical method was used in our study to identify pathological liars and to distinguish them from prolific liars (Curtis & Hart, 2020b). We used a negative binomial regression instead of using a Poisson regression due to its ability to better handle overdispersed count or rate data (Gardner et al., 1995). We also used the likelihood ratio chi-square test to examine the fit of our model of identifying pathological liars from nonpathological liars. In identifying prolific liars from within the nonpathological lying sample, a D closest to 1 led to identification of two groups: those who told zero to two lies per day and those who told three or more lies per day (prolific liars). As one can see, there are various ways that the outliers or prolific liar can be separated from the nonprolific liars.

DEMOGRAPHICS OF BIG LIARS

To understand the characteristics of people who lie a lot, we can start by examining the basic demographic traits of liars. In their large national study of liars, Patterson and Kim (1991) found that regardless of the part of the country that they examined, U.S. men lied more than U.S. women. In their national study, Serota et al. (2010), also found that men reported lying more than women, although the difference was small (men told 1.93 lies per day and women told 1.39) and not statistically significant. Other studies have reported a gender difference in the tendency to tell lies, again showing that men lie more than women (Jonason et al., 2014; Park et al., 2021; Serota & Levine, 2015). More nuanced research has found that the gender of the target of the lie matters, in that women tend to tell more altruistic lies to other women (DePaulo et al., 1993). In two large studies we have conducted, we did not find significant gender differences in lying, even when controlling for other demographic variables such as age (Hart, Beech, & Curtis, 2022; Hart, Curtis, & Randell, 2022). However, when we examined just the top 5% of liars, we did find that men made up a disproportionately large segment of that group. Where gender differences in lying do exist, this could be related to the finding that men tend to have more permissive attitudes about lying than women do (Levine et al., 1992).

There is also evidence that men and women differ in the manner in which they lie. For instance, a variety of studies have shown that women are more likely than men to tell lies aimed at benefiting another person, such as telling altruistic white lies (DePaulo et al., 1996; Erat & Gneezy, 2012; Feldman et al., 2002). Men, on the other hand, are more willing to tell self-serving lies that exact some obvious cost to the recipient. The findings that men lie more than women may result from the fact that men tend to be less bothered by lying and see lying as more acceptable (Levine et al., 1992). In a large meta-analysis examining the relationship between gender and dishonesty across 380 studies, Gerlach and colleagues (2019) found that men were more dishonest than women. However, the difference was relatively small, with men only 4% more dishonest than women. Additionally, Ning and Crossman (2007) found that women were actually more accepting of all types of lies. Thus, there is conflicting evidence about gender and lying, but it may be the case that the biggest liars tend to be men.

Age is another factor associated with lie frequency. Although lying begins at around age 2 or 3 years and quickly increases in frequency (Lee, 2000), by the time people reach their teenage years, their propensity to tell lies peaks and then begins to decrease throughout adulthood (Debey et al., 2015; Gerlach et al., 2019; Glätzle-Rützler & Lergetporer, 2015; Serota et al., 2010). Thus, all things being equal, we can conclude that teenagers and young adults will tend to be the biggest liars. Across two of our studies, the top 5% big liars had an average age 3 to 4 years younger than their typically honest counterparts (Hart, Beech, & Curtis, 2022; Hart, Curtis, & Randell, 2022). Some have suggested that younger people may lie more often because younger people are more likely to be under the oppressive control of authority figures such as parents and teachers (Jensen et al., 2004). Essentially, they argue, younger people use lying as a way to assert their autonomy. However, more recent work has found that younger people tend to lie more, even when the lies are not directed at authority figures (Warmelink, 2021). For instance, younger people are more likely to lie to spare someone's feelings or to protect someone else.

Warmelink (2021) suggested that one explanation for this age shift in lying is that older adults report that they would feel more guilty about lying than younger adults would. Researchers have also found that older adults generally hold more negative attitudes about lying than younger people (Ning & Crossman, 2007).

Social class is also associated with lying. Researchers have found that upper-class people are significantly more likely to lie and cheat than lower-class individuals (Piff et al., 2012). In a negotiation task, upper-class people were more likely to lie to advantage themselves. They were also more likely to lie in a game to get a larger cash prize. The authors concluded that positive attitudes toward greed seemed to drive the relationship between social class and lying, with upper-class individuals being more likely to endorse positive attitudes about greed. Further, they argued that upper-class people are less likely to be concerned about how others judge them (and their lying). Finally, they argued that upper-class people possess the social and material resources to deal with any negative reactions to their dishonesty. Dubois and colleagues (2015) elaborated on these findings that class differences account for why people lie. They found that upper-class people were more apt to lie in selfish ways. In contrast, lower-class people were more inclined to lie to help others altruistically. Beyond that, they found that a sense of power seemed to drive selfish lying. So, it may be that big liars are proportionally located in both upper and lower classes depending on the types of lies one is examining.

BELIEFS

Beyond simple demographics, attitudes and beliefs drive much of human behavior, including lying. For instance, religious beliefs have been examined as predictors of honesty or dishonesty. Religious people are certainly more trusted than nonreligious people (Gervais et al., 2011; Moon et al., 2018). There is some evidence that those who hold religious beliefs are less likely to endorse or see justifications for lying and may actually be less likely to lie than secular people (Oliveira & Levine, 2008; Shalvi & Leiser, 2013). However, others have failed to find evidence that religious adherents are any more honest than nonreligious people (see Kramer & Shariff, 2016, for a review). More broadly, Hofmann and colleagues (2014) studied more than 1,200 people and found no difference in any class of immoral acts including dishonesty between religious and nonreligious people. In fact, some researchers have found that people for whom religion is especially important may be even more likely to lie (Childs, 2013). Mazar and colleagues (2008) carried out a study to examine whether dishonesty would be affected by religious moral reminders. Participants were asked to recall the Ten Commandments or not and were then given the opportunity to cheat and lie. They reported that people who were given the religious moral reminder actually cheated and lied less. However, a subsequent multilab study attempted to replicate these findings using more than 4,600 participants (Verschuere et al., 2018). The researchers found that religious moral reminders did not affect honesty. These findings suggest that religiosity may not be a predictor variable of honesty. The mixed results are inconclusive and warrant more research to fully examine this area.

A set of beliefs that does seem to harmonize with a person's patterns of lying is their general attitudes about dishonesty in communication (Oliveira & Levine, 2008). The Revised Lie Acceptability Scale (Oliveira & Levine) has people indicate the degree to which they agree with statements such as "honesty is always the best policy," "it is often better to lie than to hurt someone's feelings," and "there is nothing wrong with bending the truth now and then." Those who saw lying as more acceptable tended to not be as upset when they were lied to. We conducted a study that, in part, explored how attitudes about lying are related to a person's tendency to lie. Using the Revised Lie Acceptability Scale, we found that seeing lies as acceptable (or a more favorable attitude toward lying) was one of the strongest predictors of a person's tendency to tell lies (Hart et al., 2019).

DISPOSITIONS OF LIARS

When considering people who lie prolifically, most probably consider that the liar is somehow deeply flawed at the level of their personality. Or if not flawed, at least different. Personality and dispositions can be thought of as relatively enduring characteristics of individuals that influence their thoughts, actions, and feelings. We explore several studies that have measured the degree to which various personality traits correlate with lying.

In one of our studies, we examined the degree to which the Big Five personality traits were associated with lying (Hart et al., 2019). The Big Five personality structure is a set of five basic traits factors thought to subsume all other personality traits (Costa & McCrae, 1992). The first factor, Openness, is the tendency to be imaginative, curious and attentive to feelings and to prefer variety. The next trait is Conscientiousness. It is the degree to which one is organized, focused, reliable, self-disciplined, and dutiful. Next is Extraversion, which is the disposition to enthusiastically and positively engage with others. Extraverts tend to seek out stimulation through socialization. The next trait is Agreeableness, which is a temperament marked by the pursuit of social harmony. People high in Agreeableness tend to be helpful, trustworthy, kind, and open to compromise. The final trait, Neuroticism, is a person's proneness to negative emotional instability. People who are high in Neuroticism are inclined to experience situations as stressful; are vulnerable to frustration; and react with anger, upset, and other negative emotional states. Those low in Neuroticism tend to remain calm and in good spirits, even in challenging situations.

In our study (Hart et al., 2019), we measured Big Five personality traits in 352 people and then assessed their tendency to tell self-serving lies, altruistic lies aimed at helping others, and vindictive lies told to harm or undermine others. For self-serving lies, we found that Openness, Conscientiousness, Extraversion, and Agreeableness were negatively correlated with lying, meaning that as those traits went up, self-serving lying tended to go down. On the other hand, the more neurotic someone was, the more they tended to tell self-serving lies. For altruistic lies, only Conscientiousness was correlated, such that people higher in conscientiousness told fewer altruistic lies. For vindictive lies, only Agreeableness was correlated in the expected direction; the higher a person was in Agreeableness, the less prone they were to tell vindictive lies. A large meta-analysis by Heck and colleagues (2018), found that only Agreeableness was consistently correlated with dishonesty, where more agreeable people lied less. When asking people about their own abilities to tell lies, Elaad and Reizer (2015) found that people with low levels of Conscientiousness, Agreeableness, and Neuroticism, and high levels of Openness and Extraversion reported the highest levels of lie telling ability. So, it looks like Big Five personality traits do correlate with lying, although not consistently across studies, contexts, or types of lies, but low levels of agreeableness and conscientiousness seem to be the best predictors of who will be the biggest liars.

Another proposed personality structure called the HEXACO is similar but not identical to the Big Five (Ashton et al., 2004). The biggest difference is that the HEXACO model adds a sixth factor called Honesty–Humility. It includes items such as "If I knew that I could never get caught, I would be willing to steal a million dollars" and "If I want something from someone, I will laugh at that person's worst jokes." The scale is geared toward measuring the degree to which someone is willing to manipulate others for their own gain, break rules, and feel entitled. Perhaps not surprisingly, people who score low on Honesty–Humility are more likely to lie and behave deceptively. Heck and colleagues (2018) found that Honesty–Humility "is the single most valid predictor of dishonest behavior amongst basic personality traits" (p. 365).

An additional personality feature that appears to be associated with lying is self-esteem. Self-esteem is one's subjective self-appraisal or sense of self-worth (Rosenberg, 1965). William James (1890) explained self-esteem as a consequence of the ratio of subjective successes and failures people experience in their lives. If one perceives that they are succeeding at life more than failing, their esteem is high; if not, their self-esteem is low. Low self-esteem has previously been associated with cheating and dishonesty (Lobel & Levanon, 1988; Ward, 1986), although those studies did not specifically examine lying. One study did compare the self-esteem of those people who lie at least once a day to those who do not (Grant et al., 2019). That investigation found a small difference with daily liars having lower self-esteem. We carried out our own study that examined whether the propensity to lie was associated with self-esteem (Hart et al., 2019). We found that low self-esteem was a much stronger predictor of telling self-serving and altruistic lies than any other personality trait we measured.

However, self-esteem did not significantly predict vindictive lying. There is compelling evidence that low self-esteem is associated with dishonest behavior, including lying.

Perhaps one of the most studied facets of personality associated with lying is referred to as the dark triad (Paulhus & Williams, 2002). The personality components of the dark triad are narcissism, psychopathy, and Machiavellianism. These three aversive personality traits have been lumped together because of the shared pattern of the offensive and malevolent social behaviors that accompany them. Narcissism is characterized by low levels of empathy accompanied by an egoistic sense of grandiosity and pride. People who are high in psychopathy engage in impulsive and selfish antisocial behavior, have low levels of empathy or remorse, and are thrill-seeking (Hare, 1999). Machiavellian people are manipulative and tend to callously exploit others to achieve their aims. They tend to be self-interested, cynical, and amoral in their outlook. It should come as no surprise that each of the dark triad traits is associated with dishonesty (Aghababaei et al., 2014), cheating (Esteves et al., 2021), and criminality (Edwards et al., 2017; Lyons & Jonason, 2015). There is also evidence that the traits are specifically linked to lie frequency, with narcissistic, psychopathic, and Machiavellian people lying more often (Daiku et al., 2021; Flexon et al., 2016; Halevy et al., 2014; Hart et al., 2019; Jonason et al., 2014; Zvi & Elaad, 2018). Although it may be obvious that the malevolent features of the dark triad are associated with criminal offending, there is also growing evidence that dark triad traits are beneficial in one's rise to the top in the hierarchies of the business world (Benning et al., 2018; Spurk et al., 2016). Relatedly, the nonmalevolent soft skill set of social adroitness, such as politeness, flattery, listening, adapting to different people, allows people to operate smoothly and effectively in social environments. Possession of those social tools is associated with higher rates of lying (Kashy & DePaulo, 1996). If one is searching for big liars, then exploring the dark triad is a good place to start.

Some deception researchers have also examined the role that attachment styles play in deception patterns. The concept of attachment styles is that people differ in the beliefs and expectations they have about their attachments with others, which colors the manner in which they form and maintain close relationships, with each attachment style represented by different relational characteristics (Hazan & Shaver, 1994). For instance, securely attached people are comfortable becoming emotionally close and vulnerable with others because they view others as dependable and benevolent. People with an anxious attachment style are insecure and worried about their worth in relationships. Avoidant people are untrusting and try to avoid relational intimacy. Cole (2001) found that people with anxious and avoidant attachment styles were more likely to lie to their romantic partners. He posited that people with an anxious attachment style may lie to appease their partners and avoid relational ruptures, whereas avoidantly attached people lie to avoid intimacy and maintain relational distance. Ennis and colleagues (2008) subsequently replicated the finding that anxious and avoidant attachment styles were associated with lying to romantic partners but went on to show that the same held true for lying to strangers and to nonromantic friends.

We close our summary of dispositional correlates of lying with a brief coverage of some additional traits associated with dishonesty. Cohen and colleagues (2012) found that people who are prone to guilt tend to be honest, whereas people not racked by guilt are much more willing to engage in lying and other unethical behaviors. Ashton and Lee (2007, 2008, 2009) also found guilt-proneness positively correlated with honesty. Eswara and Suryarekha (1974) found that people who are less anxious are more inclined to lie. Gino and Ariely (2012) found that creative people are more likely to lie, concluding that creativity is important in fabricating falsehoods.

Researchers have also examined the relationship between intelligence and lying, but findings have been mixed. Sarzyńska and colleagues (2017) found that people who score higher in intelligence were more likely to lie to earn money. In contrast, Littrell and colleagues (2021) found that the tendency to lie was negatively correlated (although not significantly so) with cognitive ability. Pauls and Crost (2005) found that people with higher cognitive ability are more believable liars. However, Wright and colleagues

(2013) examined whether lying ability was associated with general intelligence and found no such correlation. Likewise, Grant and colleagues (2019) found that more frequent liars were no different in cognitive functioning than more honest people. Thus, there is no clear relationship between dishonesty and intelligence.

POWER OF THE SITUATION

There is a certain appeal to the idea that personality drives honesty and dishonesty. If one only understood the nature of someone's personality, then whether they could be trusted could be assessed. However, decades of psychological research have made clear that situational factors interact with and often have a far greater influence than personality on behavioral outcomes (Buss, 1977; Kenrick & Funder, 1988; Mischel, 1968). When it comes to lying, the role of situational variables appears to be key. Deception researcher Dan Ariely said, "One of the frightening conclusions we have is that what separates honest people from not-honest people is not necessarily character, it's opportunity" (Vedantam, 2018, para. 4).

The idea that lying is situational is not new (Bok, 1978, Levine, 2020; McCornack et al., 2014; Vrij, 2008). Even a review of nonscientific literature indicates that the nature of humans is not to lie always or even to lie randomly. Rather, people selectively lie when the situation presents a set of circumstances and incentives for which lying appears to be a more preferential strategy than telling the truth (Bond et al., 2013; Levine, 2020). Simple economic models would suggest that people would likely be more inclined to lie when the risk is low and the rewards are high. A large meta-analysis examined this role of rewards and found that people are significantly more likely to be dishonest when the potential reward from lying is high (Gerlach et al., 2019). Likewise, the perceived risk of getting caught influences the likelihood of lying. People lie when there is a better chance of it going undetected (Lundquist et al., 2009; Markowitz & Levine, 2021). Being able to get away with a lie predicts deception more accurately than personality does. Researchers have examined the influence that various situational factors such as moral appeals, information about social norms, and threats of punishment have on dishonesty. Threats seem to have the biggest influence of all (Fellner et al., 2013).

Aside from simple risk and reward variables, over the past few decades, researchers have elucidated many other situational contours that seem to give rise to lying. Some situational variables seem fairly mundane on their surface yet have surprisingly potent effects on the tendency to deceive. Zhong and colleagues (2010) found that the lighting in a room influenced lying. Specifically, when the room was darker, people were more likely to lie to secure money than when the room was brightly lit. The researchers argued that the sense of anonymity conferred by darkness is what drove the lying. Time of day also seems to be an important factor in honesty and dishonesty. Kouchaki and Smith (2014) conducted a series of studies in which they found that people are significantly more likely to lie and otherwise behave dishonestly in the afternoon compared with the morning. They found that people tend to be more morally engaged at the start of the day, but that moral engagement fades throughout the day.

This idea that active engagement ebbs and flows has been studied more broadly. Roy Baumeister and his colleagues (1998) argued that self-control and willpower are effortful to exercise. They postulated that if people work too hard for too long at controlling themselves, then eventually they are taxed to their limits, what they called *ego depletion*. Ego-depletion theory posits that if a person depletes his or her ego in one self-control task, then they will be unable to exercise self-control in other, unrelated efforts. Gino and colleagues (2011) examined whether ego depletion would influence one's ability to be honest. They had participants complete a demanding task that required vigilant inhibition of certain responses, thus, presumably depleting the egos of the participants. Next, participants were placed in a situation in which they could earn more money by lying. The researchers found that, indeed, ego-depleted people were more likely to lie. The researchers provided evidence that the lying was partly due to the ego-depletion task impairing people's ability to consider morality. Consistent with this ego-depletion model, some research found that fatigue caused by a lack of sleep increased the odds of lying (Barnes et al., 2011).

Other researchers have studied the effects of moral reminders on lying. If college students were required to sign a statement indicating they understood that lying, cheating, and other forms of dishonesty were considered violations of the university's honor code, the students were significantly less likely to lie afterward (Mazar et al., 2008). In a similar vein of moral reflection, another study found that if people sat in front of a mirror where they could see themselves, they were less likely to lie for money (Gino & Mogilner, 2014). The researchers contended that when people are forced to self-reflect and evaluate themselves, they are less likely to engage in behavior for which they would judge themselves harshly. As mentioned previously, despite widespread coverage of reports that thinking about the Ten Commandments reduces lying (Mazar et al., 2008), many other researchers have failed to replicate that finding (Verschuere et al., 2018).

As social animals, perhaps it should not be surprising that interactions with others can influence one's likelihood of lying. For instance, seeing others lie can influence people to lie. Ariely (2012) reported that if a person from the same college appeared to lie, other students from that school would follow suit and lie as well. However, if the first liar wore a sweatshirt indicating that they were from a rival university, students were less likely to follow their lead. Thus, a model can draw people into dishonesty, but more so if that model is seen as one of their own. Feeling connected to the liar model seems to be important in the power of influence. Gino and Galinsky (2012) found that even sharing the same birthday is enough of a connection to provide this influence. The link between social connection and lying is not that simple, however. Research has indicated different results related to telling lies in various relationships. Some findings suggest that people tell fewer lies to those who are emotionally close, telling fewer self-serving lies but more other-oriented lies to their partner (DePaulo & Kashy, 1998), whereas other studies report more lies are told to those who are emotionally close (e.g., family and friends) than to strangers (Serota et al., 2010; Serota & Levine, 2015). Yet other findings show no difference related to relationship type (Dunbar & Johnson, 2015). Some research has addressed how the locus of orientation—whether the lie is told for the teller or receiver—is responsible for relational results. For example, people are much more likely to tell self-serving lies to strangers than to people whom they consider close (Whitty & Carville, 2008). When it comes to other-oriented lies (e.g., lies aimed at protecting another's dignity), people are more likely to tell them to people they are closer to than strangers. Ackert and colleagues (2011) also found social distance can affect the likelihood of lying. They argued that people have concerns about what other people think about them. This is especially true as people increase in their social closeness, which breeds feelings of psychological closeness (e.g., familiarity and intimacy). When closeness is high, people are more inclined to lie to preserve their self-image or protect others. The researchers argued that this is because people feel more compelled to manage other's impressions when a high degree of psychological closeness exists.

More broadly, Mann and colleagues (2014) offered evidence that lying is socially transmitted through social groups. They found that whether one lies a lot or very little is tied to with whom they affiliate: Liars socialize with liars, and honest people socialize with honest people. They found this in biologically related groups but also in nonrelated groups.

All manner of dishonesty, cheating, and other corrupt behavior emerges from groups and organizations, so researchers have examined the role of group dynamics in dishonesty. Cohen and colleagues (2010) have made clear that groups are greedier than the individuals who compose those groups. Cohen et al. (2009) found that people in groups are more likely to lie when deception confers a strategic advantage. However, they are also more likely to be honest than individuals when honesty confers an advantage, so it may simply be that groups operate in a more strategically effective way than individuals. Kocher and colleagues (2018) also found that individuals shift to more dishonest thought patterns when they begin to work in a group. When individuals form into groups, they collectively are able to formulate more arguments for why lying is morally defensible. Additionally, the diffusion of moral responsibility across all of the group members leaves any single member feeling less personally responsible for the dishonesty of the group.

Social interactions often give rise to emotional changes, and as it turns out, these emotional changes influence lying. Yip and Schweitzer (2016) carried out a series of studies in which they induced anger in their participants by having a confederate provide scathing feedback about an essay they had written. Shortly thereafter, in an unrelated situation, the still-angered participants were much more likely to lie to someone. The researchers went on to demonstrate that when participants were angry, it lowered their empathy toward others, which set the stage for them to lie. Interestingly, other negative emotions such as sadness did not influence lying. Yip and Schweitzer, along with others (e.g., Tangney et al., 2007), have suggested that negative emotions that leave people feeling threatened will increase lying. On the other hand, DeSteno and colleagues (2019) found that people who were placed in situations that made them feel happy or grateful lied less.

Time pressure influences lying too. Lying takes time and effort, and there is some evidence that our default position is to tell the truth (Foerster et al., 2013; Levine, 2020). There is evidence that when people are under extreme time pressure to respond, they are apt to respond with the truth. However, if there is time to deliberate, people consider lying, and sometimes do. This finding seems at odds with previously discussed research in which people are less likely to lie when they consider the moral implications. Perhaps people tend to lie when they have time to think about whether they can get away with it, or when they have time to morally justify it. Or it may simply be that some complex lying takes time, and when a person has no time, she or he may just be honest.

The search for big liars grows complicated when the notion that much lying is situationally influenced is considered. Rather than thinking of big liars as a type of person, people who tell numerous lies may be considered within their larger social environments. As the field of psychology and psychopathology has indicated with regard to most behavior, lying is the result of an interplay between situational and personality variables. Lying can be understood by the person and the environment, nature and nurture, diathesis and stress, and many levels of analysis (biopsychosocial models).

SUMMARY OF THOUGHTS ON FREQUENT LYING

Most would not choose to affiliate with people who lie frequently. People generally do not like to be lied to; they experience it as aversive and hold many negative attitudes toward those who lie (Curtis, 2015; Curtis & Dickens, 2017; Curtis & Hart, 2015; Curtis et al., 2018; Kowalski et al., 2003). They view it as a betrayal. Liars have the effect of fracturing the trust that serves as the glue for societies (Bok, 1978; Harris, 2013). Frequent deception is toxic for relationships, dissolving trust and intimacy (DePaulo & Kashy, 1998; DePaulo et al., 1996; Schweitzer et al., 2006) and decreasing overall relationship satisfaction (Cargill & Curtis, 2017; C. Peterson, 1996). Perhaps not surprisingly, people who lie a lot are significantly more likely to be dumped because of their lying and they are more likely to be fired or reprimanded at work because of their lying (Serota & Levine, 2015). But not all frequent liars do so for malicious reasons, and their lies may not arise from any conscious intent (McCornack et al., 2014).

Con artists, fraudsters, and scammers are people who willfully plan and execute harmful lying on a regular basis (Konnikova, 2016). Their aims are to take advantage for their own gain. Most prolific liars seem to lie frequently for more banal reasons, such as avoiding embarrassment, avoiding awkwardness, and concealing their minor shortcomings. Perhaps it is incorrect to think of frequent liars as necessarily evil or morally bankrupt people. It may be more accurate to conceptualize them simply as people whose histories, personality traits, and situational particulars place them regularly in predicaments in which they find telling the truth to be challenging. Likewise, we can view pathological liars as a subset of these frequent liars. A subset, rather than relishing their dishonesty, find their frequent lying to be a scourge, upending important facets of their lives and leaving them in continuous distress. In the next chapter, cases of these individuals are explored, followed by a discussion of the research that corroborates the idea that pathological liars suffer from their lies and have impaired functioning.

4

Case Studies of Pathological Liars

He who permits himself to tell a lie once finds it much easier to do it a second
and third time, till at length it becomes habitual.

—Thomas Jefferson (1785)

The following is a quote from a psychiatric session with a 17-year-old young man diagnosed with pathological lying (Gogineni & Newmark, 2014):

> I made a Halloween house to scare others. The visitors were frightened by falling into a trap. They would see people without limbs or dead people with their heads half sliced open. Blood was spurting on them. There was also a person hanging from a tree during the ride. If they touched anything they would be electrocuted. Zombies were present . . . and this was so frightening the police were called. This haunted house was in a field my family owned. When the police came

https://doi.org/10.1037/0000305-004
Pathological Lying: Theory, Research, and Practice, by D. A. Curtis and C. L. Hart

I took off in a red car at 400 mph and flew over a lake to escape the cops. May have been going only 100 mph. (p. 451)

It is a good practice to carefully observe a phenomenon before attempting to explain, predict, or control it. Davison and Lazarus (2007) stated that "major clinical discoveries are usually made by clinicians and then investigated by more experimentally minded workers whose subsequent findings may persuade others that a technique is worth a closer look" (p. 149). In fact, it was in reviewing some of these cases that prompted our empirical investigations and helped shape our definition of pathological lying, which is discussed further in the next chapter. In this vein, we present numerous case studies that may prove useful in helping the reader develop a sense of how pathological liars present clinically. These case studies span a century of psychological and psychiatric research and offer a breadth of exemplars. One should remain mindful that the case studies that find their way into the published literature may not be typical or representative; they may represent the extreme or unusual presentations of pathological lying, so far a departure from the norm that they draw the curiosity and attention of the people who treat them.

We first give accounts of two previously unpublished cases personally observed by one of the authors. The first case is that of Mr. L, who was first observed as an adolescent. Aside from his parents divorcing at an early age, he experienced a fairly normal and stable childhood and development. He was an extremely gregarious person with several friends, had occasional girlfriends, and had a good relationship with his family. He performed somewhat below average in school, which was attributed to a lack of interest and focus rather than cognitive deficits. Collateral information indicated that Mr. L was prone to tell many stories that seemed wildly embellished or wholly fabricated. Often the stories were fantastical accounts that presented him as extremely daring, brave, or fortunate. Examples included tales of motorcycle jumps and crashes that defied physics or human ability, stories of being pursued by and escaping from nefarious characters who intended him harm, and tales of outrageous sexual exploits in which he demonstrated remarkable sexual prowess with numerous beautiful women. By all accounts, these stories were not true. After high school, Mr. L enlisted in the army. In a conversation with one of the authors about his experiences in military basic training, Mr. L told of how he blew up a tank with a hand grenade, but nobody ever found out about it. He also gave an account of how, during firearms training, the person standing right next to him accidentally blew his head off with a gun. When it was suggested that his stories might be exaggerations, Mr. L would sometimes double-down in an effort to have the stories believed, but other times, he would acknowledge that he was merely trying to see if people would believe his outlandish story. Although he lied frequently, his lies were never directly used to exploit people financially or other-wise. Mr. L seemed to relish telling his fantastical tales, and other than having a solid reputation as a fabricator, which likely adversely affected his ability to form and maintain some relationships, he was able to maintain some relationships and maintain employment, at least during the period of observation.

The second case is that of an undergraduate university student. Mr. D was approximately 40 years old and was attending school for a midlife career change. Mr. D quickly came to the attention of numerous faculty members because of his boisterous personality and his tendency to lie in most conversations. He claimed at various times to be a Vietnam War veteran, despite being far too young for that to be true. He also claimed to have been in the special forces, yet was unable to provide any specific details about his service when asked. He claimed to have been shot multiple times, yet the story of how and when he was allegedly shot changed with each telling. He used a wheelchair and once claimed to be paralyzed yet was subsequently seen walking unassisted. He also reported to various people that he was dying from terminal brain cancer, yet that seemed to be a complete fabrication as well. His stories all seemed possible, but not very plausible. Each of his stories placed him as either a victim of bad circum-stances or as an extraordinarily capable person. Eventually, his chronic lying and other aversive personality traits led to a suggestion from univer-sity staff that he should find a different degree program to pursue. Mr. D's habit of lying seemed to significantly interfere with his ability to form or maintain social relationships and to navigate school life effectively.

EARLY CASE STUDIES

The first published case study focusing on pathological lying was written in 1891 by the German psychiatrist Anton Delbrück. He described a small group of cases of individuals who were being treated in his psychiatric hospital in part because of their extensive lying, what he termed *pseudologia fantastica* (summarized in English in Healy & Healy, 1915). The first case he described was that of a maid-servant from Austria who had traveled through Switzerland and Austria, taking on numerous identities. At various times she had convinced people that she was a wealthy friend of the bishop, an impoverished medical student, a Romanian princess, and a Spanish royal. She had forged letters from the cardinal to herself. She had disguised herself as a man and attended an educational institution until her sex was discovered, at which point she fled. Delbrück noted that this woman's lies had a hypnotic or dreamlike quality to them. She seemed to lie almost instinctively and appeared to half believe her own lies sometimes. Delbrück mused about whether her lying might be mixed with delusions. He noted that her lying was very imaginative and tended to have a boastful quality.

His second case was a woman who would regularly approach strangers and claim to be their relative visiting from another city. In cases where she managed to convince people of their familial bond, she would take up residence in their homes until she wore out her welcome. At that point, she would leave, stealing many of their belongings on her way out the door. Consequently, the woman had been imprisoned numerous times. Delbrück found that this woman would suffer from seizures followed by a delirious twilight state. While superficially her deceptive scams seemed skillful and cunning, Delbrück dug a bit deeper and found that she was no criminal mastermind. Many of the items she would steal were effectively useless to her. She would also order goods under an assumed name but never return to collect them. Delbrück noted that her ruses generally involved her attempts to portray herself as wealthier and more influential than she truly was, but he questioned whether she was indeed culpable for her dishonesty.

Delbrück's third case was that of a young man who had studied theology and was pursuing a career as a preacher. As a youth, the person had been noted as being honest. However, shortly after he had completed his theological training, the man began a habit of lying. He lied to relatives and friends about promising career offers that were coming his way. He would then borrow money from them, which they freely gave him under the belief that his career was taking off. Delbrück viewed the cases as a complex mix of delusions and deception.

His next case was a young man who appeared to have been lying excessively since childhood. He was described as artful, arrogant, and clever. In addition to lying, he frequently stole things. He began college but was sent home after just a few months, having racked up a considerable debt. By the time Delbrück saw him, the pathological liar had been an opium user for years.

In Delbrück's analysis, the pathological liars mixed lying with mistakes and perhaps delusions; their lies, however, reached pathological levels and were a cardinal feature of their presentations. He also described that their lies seemed to be manufactured in the same manner that a poet creates prose. That is, the liars wove together elaborate tales with an imaginative zeal and artistic flair.

Soon after Delbrück's publication, Köppen (1898; as translated by Healy & Healy, 1915) provided another set of case studies. Köppen noted that the lies told by pathological liars were no different in content or form than the lies told by the typical person. The lies did not seem to be delusional statements. He asserted that the lies were active fabrications that seemed to take hold of the liars such that the liar no longer had control over them. Across three cases, he described individuals who seemed to have comorbid mental health problems. Each of these individuals concocted elaborate lies that presented themselves in a much more favorable light than their actual situations would allow. Köppen also noted that in each case it was not clear that the patients were always able to clearly distinguish their concocted stories from reality.

Bernard Risch (1908, translated by Healy & Healy, 1915) reported some additional cases of pathological lying. He noted that in each case, the liar seemed to concoct stories in the same manner that a fiction writer would, creating tales of elaborate romances and fantasies. He submitted that what separated pathological liars from fiction writers was the irrepressible, egocentric desire to play the role of or become the central character in the story. His case studies detailed a man who wove together fantastical tales of adventure, hair-raising escapes from dangerous predicaments, and torrid love affairs, all of which were entirely made up. He reportedly lied continuously and derived great satisfaction out of sharing his elaborate lies with others. In another case, a man with a criminal history would concoct riveting and sensational stories of crimes he had not actually committed. He centered himself as the central heroic figure in these falsehoods.

In these early case studies of pathological lying, there is a clear selection bias. The people writing them were psychiatrists employed at asylums, so, naturally, the only pathological liars to come before them were people with rather severe psychiatric conditions. It may have been the case that many more pathological liars who lacked severe concomitant psychopathologies existed outside the walls of the institutions.

Healy and Healy (1915) personally documented a great number of cases of pathological liars in the United States. The following is one case that they considered a classic example of a pathological liar. It is the case of a 27-year-old woman named Inez who presented herself as a 17-year-old and traveled around taking advantage of others' sympathy. Despite a tremendous effort to discern the truth about Inez's life, she had spun such a web of lies that few people who had interacted with her were able to provide any reliably accurate details of who she actually was. What could be corroborated was that she moved from home to home and town to town presenting herself as a strong young woman with noble bearing and intentions who merely needed a bit of help. Families would take her in, but eventually her persistent lying would undermine any goodwill, and she would have to leave, often taking items from her hosts as she departed. The Healys studied her extensively and noted that she was a reliable reporter except when asked about the details of her own life. That is, she did not lie randomly or universally, but only when the topic was herself. The Healys wrote of her:

> In summarizing the characteristics of this woman we may first insist that she has ambition, push, and energy in high degree. Her personality as expressed in general bearing, features, and facial action is remarkably strong and convincing.... Usually Inez shows a very even temper.... Some pathological liars may be weak in character, but not Inez. She is the firmest of persons. On occasions her attitude is entirely that of the grand lady. Her type of lying is clearly pathological. It would often be very hard to discern a purpose in it, and over and over again she has defeated her own ends by further indulgence in prevarications. To her, the utterance of lies comes just as quickly and naturally as speaking the truth comes to other people. Even in interviews with us when she was voluntarily acknowledging her shortcomings in this direction she went on in the same breath to further falsifications.... The bearing of this case on the problems of testimony is interesting. As shown in our account of tests done, when objective concrete material was considered by this woman she reported it well. It is only when her egocentrism is brought into play that she becomes so definitely unreliable. This is a line of demarcation that students of this subject would do well to recognize.... Her facility with language marks her as possessing one of the chief characteristics of the pathological liar. Added to this she showed the other personal traits which we have described in detail, leading to her success in misrepresenting herself.... Her forceful personality carries her into situations which she is incompetent to live up to. The immediate way out is by creating a new complication, and this may be through lies or the simulation of illness, at which she has become an adept. Altogether, Inez must be thought of as one who is trying to satisfy certain wishes and ambitions which are too much for her resources. Towards the goal to which her nature urges her she follows the path of least resistance. Being the personality that she is, the social world offers her stimulation which does not come to others. To discuss the problem of her responsibility would be to introduce metaphysics—it is sure that in the ordinary sense she is not insane. (pp. 78–79)

The Healys went on to comment that Inez was quite intelligent. She was capable of fooling most people for a time, even the Healys who at the time were deeply involved in the study of pathological liars. Thus, unlike the earlier case studies, Inez came across as not having any obvious mental defect apart from her lying. The Healys also concluded that many of her lies were told simply because she needed to cover previous lies, suggesting that the road to pathological lying may be the proverbial slippery slope.

When analyzing the themes that occurred across all of their case studies of pathological lying, the Healys observed that a key characteristic was deep-seated egocentrism. The pathological liars almost universally spun stories about themselves, often painting themselves as heroic figures or tragic victims. They also noted that the pathological liars usually expressed little concern or sympathy for others. Furthermore, the liars seemed unable to fully appreciate how their lying negatively affected the impressions others formed of them.

A synthesis of the early pathological lying cases suggests the obvious key feature of unusually frequent displays of lying (Healy & Healy, 1915; Treanor, 2012). Often, the nature of the lies was fantastical and imaginative with some seemingly truthful yet improbable elements woven in. The lies tended to paint the patient in a positive light, and their motivation was often not rooted in any obvious gain for the liar, but rather for some vague self-promotion. Helene Deutsch (Deutsch & Roazen, 1922/1982) noted that the lies often had a daydream quality about them. In fact, she posited that pseudologia fantastica (fantasy lies) were actually the same as the daydreams that most people have, representing their dreams and longings. She argued that the difference is that most people keep their daydream fantasies to themselves out of shame, whereas the pseudologue presents their fantasies to others as if they were realities.

In 1933, Dirk Wiersma published several case studies describing pathological lying. In his report, he noted some defining characteristics. In one case that he considered a true example of pathological lying, he described a young adult man who was institutionalized after the judge in his theft case found him quite odd. The psychiatrist, Wiersma, gave an account of the young man's claims, which included elaborate stories of traveling to

Spain, befriending royalty, and living in a castle. He also described friendships he had made with German aristocrats. Wiersma noted that these stories did not seem to be delusions but rather fantasy tales that the patient recognized and would sometimes acknowledge were not entirely true. The patient eventually shifted from lies that were fantastical and romantic to those that were more mundane, if somewhat adventurous. With all of the lies, the patient was thought to lie because he was emotionally captivated by his tales and did not really seem to care about whether they were truthful. He did not lie to exploit others but rather to entertain himself.

By contrast, Wiersma presented a second case of an individual who lied with great frequency but who seemed to do so only when the deception provided an opportunity to take advantage of someone. The patient marveled at how easy it was to dupe most of the gullible populace. Once placed in the asylum, with no opportunities to use deceit for his personal gain, his lying stopped almost entirely. Wiersma argued that this person was not a pathological liar, but merely a criminal. The key distinction as he saw it was that a mere criminal liar is always keenly aware that they are lying and only lies when it promises to be a profitable enterprise. Pathological liars, on the other hand, do not always seem to notice when they are lying and do so for nonexploitive reasons.

In a third case, Wiersma described a young man who also lied extraordinarily. This patient, although occasionally involved in criminality, did not lie principally for financial gain. Instead, he made boisterous, untrue claims about his accomplishments, position in life, and abilities. His lies seemed focused on presenting himself as more capable, interesting, and accomplished than he actually was. This patient, unlike Wiersma's first patient, seemed always fully aware of when he was lying and when he was being truthful. The patient also seemed to be aware of his own motivations to lie, telling Wiersma that he lied to seem more important or interesting to others. Thus, vanity and ambition appeared to drive his deception.

On the basis of the three cases, Wiersma identified three categories of people who lie excessively. First, there are normal liars whose sole purpose in lying is to gain an advantage or avoid punishment. They lie to exploit others or to avoid detection for primarily financial, material, or nonmaterial social gains. Criminals would fall into the normal liar category. These people regularly scheme to swindle people, so lying, being a primary tool of their criminal enterprise, is used frequently.

Second, there are pathological liars. These individuals lie regularly but do not seem to do so because of any rational motives, such as tangible rewards or avoidance of punishment. Instead, the lie itself seems to be rewarding. The excitement of presenting a fictional version of oneself, especially one in which the liar is exceptional, motivates the pathological liar. Pathological liars often appear to discern when they are shifting between truth and lie. Their lies give the impression of being designed to create fantastical autobiographical narratives, devoid of any intention to secure tangible gains. It is as if the lies are aimed at escaping the prosaic reality of their true selves.

Finally, Wiersma opined, there are liars with pseudologia fantastica (aka mythomania). These individuals possess the same features of the pathological liar but seem to slip from truth to lie without being aware of or having a care about the distinction. Their lies take on a daydream quality. Although they may have the ability to acknowledge their deception when it is forcefully brought to their attention, they seem to have little concern about having their lies detected.

Rather than viewing the three types of frequent liars as categorically different, Wiersma concluded that these types exist along a continuum. They all seem to lie, but the lies move from rationally motivated on one end of the continuum to largely irrational on the other end. The psychological features that seemed to be associated with movement toward the pseudologia fantastica end of the continuum were, according to Wiersma, vanity, a nervous temperament, and an infantile character.

MODERN ANALYSES OF CASE STUDIES

After Wiersma's 1933 review of cases of pathological lying, the next such review was not published for more than 50 years (B. H. King & Ford, 1988). B. H. King and Ford (1988) analyzed 72 historical case studies of pathological liars. They asserted that the key features of pathological liars were that they told lies that were not entirely improbable (but perhaps implausible), their lies were maintained over time, the liars recognized the falsity of their claims, and the lies seemed intended to self-aggrandize rather than to generate a tangible profit. B. H. King and Ford also summarized the common features of the pathological liars, although they cautioned readers that the published case studies are likely a biased selection of highly interesting cases that managed to draw the attention of treating psychiatrists. The cases were equally likely to be men or women. The case studies tended to report patients who were in early adulthood, although the lying tended to begin in adolescence. The patients were of average to slightly below average intelligence. A substantial portion had evidence of neurological problems such as epilepsy. They also had a higher than usual incidence of life adjustment problems such as criminal arrests and institutionalization.

In one of the largest recent reviews of pathological lying case studies, Treanor (2012) noted that the case literature was inconsistent and unconvincing in drawing distinctions among pathological lying, pseudologia fantastica, or any other terms used to describe people who lie in a pathological manner. She observed that across case studies spanning a century, various terms had been used, and their meanings were construed inconsistently. She noted that it was nearly impossible even to identify a consensus perspective of what the key traits of pathological lying were or how the disorder should be defined.

To discern what the principal traits of pathological lying were, Treanor (2012) tabulated basic details from all of the historical cases she could locate and then carried out an in-depth thematic analysis in an attempt to identify features that were common across all or most pathological lying case studies. She located 132 case studies for her analysis. She decided not to include cases for which there was no English translation, the patient was a young child, there was insufficient detail for the analysis, the presentation was starkly different from the current understanding of pathological lying, or in which the lying could be better explained by psychosis or delusional disorder. She was left with 64 complete case studies that met the criteria for her analysis. The mean age of the cases was 24 years with a median of 20. The gender split was fairly even with 55% of the cases being men and 45% women. Her analysis revealed a great many symptoms and features that were present in only one or a handful of cases, suggesting that presentations of pathological lying can vary considerably. However, Treanor was able to identify several features that were common among most, but not all, cases: The lies described humanly possible events, the person had been exhibiting problematic lying for years, the person lied frequently, the person was aware that they were lying, the lies were self-aggrandizing, the lies often had themes of heroism or victimization, and the lying often did not seem to be motivated by any obvious purpose or gain.

PLAUSIBILITY OF THE LIES

In her analysis, Treanor (2012) found that for the great majority of cases (more than 98%), the person told lies that described circumstances that, although perhaps unlikely, were at least within the realm of the possible. We have also found this pattern in our own review of historical case studies. For example, in a recently published case study, Frierson and Joshi (2018) reported the following:

> During his initial presentation, he gave a history of numerous events in his life which appeared unusual to the point of being unbelievable, and therefore their validity was suspect. The defendant claimed that he was kidnapped by a Mexican drug cartel when he was four years old. He reported that he was eventually rescued by "biker gangs" and his family was placed in the witness protection program. The defendant stated that he directly witnessed a cousin kill himself by shooting himself in the head. His mother reported that all of these claims were untrue and that he had never been kidnapped or placed in a witness protection program. She reported that his cousin did commit suicide, but it was not witnessed by the defendant. He reported that he had a high school diploma from a prestigious high school. He reported that he made the highest score possible on the Armed Services Vocational Aptitude Battery (ASVAB). The defendant claimed that he was in the US Army for six and a half years. During his time in

the Army, he stated that he was a Nuclear, Biological, and Chemical Operations Specialist. He reported that he later became a member of numerous Army Special Forces (Delta Forces, Green Beret, and part of Black Operations). He alleged that he was in situations where he saw people get killed in combat. The defendant's family reported that he did not graduate from high school, but he did obtain a GED. His family reported that he was not in the military for six and a half years (he was in for much less). His family also reported that he was not involved in active combat and was not in Special Forces, but he did score very high on the ASVAB and was a Nuclear, Biological, and Chemical Operations Specialist. (p. 977)

However, in other cases, we have found that the liar may report events that are inconsistent with the realm of possible events. In some cases, this may simply be due to the liar's ignorance about the nature of reality. An example may be seen in the case report of a patient in Mitchell and Francis (2003):

While undergoing residential treatment, he was referred for a psychological evaluation due to apparent exaggeration of his alcohol use history. During the evaluation, he described a history of alcohol use that defied biological possibility for an individual of his height and weight. . . . Laboratory tests sensitive to heavy drinking were within the normal range and collateral information suggested a remote history of minor abusive drinking. . . . The history that emerged from his parents and other collateral sources indicated that he was an individual with low intellectual functioning. (p. 188)

Although more rare, we have also located cases studies in which the pathological liar's claims seem wholly unbelievable. For example,

Once I saved a friend of mine. To help this friend I had to jump 1 mile up from a helicopter into a pool of alligators and sharks in Florida. I was able to fend off the shark attack and outmuscle the alligators with my strength. My friend treated me like I was a hero. And I had to use a harpoon to kill the many sharks and gators. The harpoon went into the alligator's eyeball. (Gogineni & Newmark, 2014, p. 451)

CHRONICITY

In the majority of case studies, the authors note that the problematic lying had occurred for years, often beginning in childhood. We have found consistent evidence that the pervasive lying seems to begin early in life, where extensive histories are described. For instance,

> His mother noted behavioural problems from an early age, including lying and frequent theft from the home. At the age of 11 he was sent to a boarding school for maladjusted children where problems of lying and a disregard for the property of others continued. He was not thought to be educationally subnormal, but had difficulties in learning to read and write which were attributed to poor concentration and his disturbed behaviour. (Sharrock & Cresswell, 1989, p. 324)

Here is another example from Hardie and Reed (1998):

> His mother stated that he had told untruths from the age of 11. During his teenage years he would frequently lie about trivial day-to-day occurrences, which offered him no apparent gain. This continued into adult life and was a prominent feature of his behaviour when with his parents between prison sentences and hospital admissions. (p. 199)

FREQUENCY

A key feature of most definitions of pathological lying is that the person lies often. In the majority of case studies, this theme of frequent prevarication is indicated. In her analysis, Treanor (2012) found that high frequency was explicitly mentioned in 80% of the cases. The remaining cases did not mention the frequency of lying, but the reports also did not contradict the theme of frequent lying. An example of such frequency evidence in the case study literature includes the following:

> The individual in question was a 20-year-old white Canadian male. He had been committed to the provincial penitentiary for a series of relatively minor offenses and had earlier absconded from a remand center. He caused concern to both the prison staff and the parole

board because of his tendency to make statements that, upon check, proved to be false (it must be stressed that this tendency was felt to be markedly more pronounced than is typical among prisoners). (Stones, 1976, pp. 219–220)

High-frequency lying is clearly demonstrated in the following case report. All of the claims made by the individual occurred during a brief hospital intake interview. Collateral reports subsequently indicated that all of the claims were massive distortions or outright lies:

The patient mentioned that he had been struggling with sadness and suicidality since his pregnant fiancée had recently been killed in an automobile accident. . . . He reported that he was engaged to be married and worked as a mathematics and physics professor at a prestigious university as well as an engineering consultant in the private sector. He also reported that he had sustained a number of musculoskeletal injuries resulting in chronic pain while playing Division I football in college and that he had been drafted by the National Football League. . . . Reporting that he had been suffering from very low mood since his pregnant fiancée had been killed by a drunk driver eight months ago. Because the electronic medical record indicated that he had been engaged to be married just one month ago, we asked him to confirm the date of his fiancée's death, which he could not recall. . . . He spoke about his profession as a tenured mathematics and physics professor at a prestigious university although when asked about the nature of his research he could only vaguely describe studying "time bends in space using some of Einstein's old formulae. . . ." When asked to provide a collateral contact, he reported that both of his parents, multiple siblings, and cousins had died during his early childhood. (Thom et al., 2017, pp. 1–2)

As another example, H. Green et al. (1999) reported the following collateral report about a pathological liar:

Information obtained subsequently from a close family member revealed a different story with a long history of deception ("she was always lying"; "I would go so far to say that she didn't know how to tell the truth"). (p. 255)

A review of case studies, old and recent, supports the notion that a key characteristic of pathological lying is a statistically anomalous amount of lying.

AWARENESS OF THE LIE

Another theme Treanor (2012) extracted was that the pathological liars knew that they were lying. That is, when pressed, many of the individuals acknowledged that what they had said was factually incorrect. This finding is important because disagreements over whether pathological liars know they are lying or not appear in the historical literature. Treanor found that in 56% of cases, there were indications that the person was aware they were lying, in 41% there was no mention, and in only 3% of cases the liar seemed unable to recognize that they were lying. For instance, in Mitchell and Francis (2003), the authors made clear that the pathological liar was aware of his deception:

> He was interviewed a second time and gently confronted with various discrepancies between his self-report and available fact. He initially attempted to provide more elaborate fabrications to account for prior inconsistencies then admitted that his fabrications were fantasies that he had repeated to peers in order earn their respect and thereby become more compatible with others. . . . He was discharged from treatment, but not before he was observed telling additional fabrications about his background to other staff and patients. (p. 188)

In their recent case report, Frierson and Joshi (2018) also noted that the liar was aware of his deceit:

> He demonstrated that he could back down from his assertions when faced with alternative collateral information. After being confronted about his electrical company not existing, he finally admitted that it was aspirational though not operational, but that he had obtained a business identification number, and the persons he said worked for him had agreed to come to and work for the company. He admitted that there was not a large million dollar contract with a local

university. This was quite different than how he initially presented this information—that the company existed and had been awarded a $1.7 million contract. (p. 978)

In other cases, however, awareness is much less clear, making it challenging to determine if one is observing lies or delusions. For example,

> The unit staff pointed out he often makes things up about himself in the middle of a conversation, usually if it serves to elevate his status or reputation. It is really difficult to tell if he is doing this consciously or not though. I am giving him the benefit of the doubt at this point in treating him as delusional, but it could be pseudologia fantastica or some other component of narcissistic personality disorder. (Frierson & Joshi, 2018, p. 978)

SELF-AGGRANDIZING

Another regular theme in pathological cases is that the lies are not random in their focus. Rather, they are often tales that paint the liar in a positive light. The lies frequently portray the liar as possessing an impressive set of abilities, holding high-status positions, or accomplishing feats that few mere mortals could pull off. For instance, consider the following case from Newmark et al. (1999):

> Finally, the patient's stories had a self-aggrandizing quality. He described himself as having several prestigious positions and roles. . . . Despite reports of the patient being a noncombat veteran, he allegedly reported serving as a Green Beret and working for the CIA for 37 years. He also claimed that he was a martial arts expert. . . . He made allusions to involvement in multiple covert operations. He claimed that he was trained to speak Spanish, Korean, German, and Russian. (pp. 91–92)

Here is another example from Hardie and Reed (1998):

> He had been pretending to be a doctor in three separate hospitals. . . . He had wandered the wards as a doctor, talked to patients and relatives,

and on one occasion joined a teaching round for medical students. This was the latest of a series of similar offences for which the modus operandi was the same. . . . He was attempting to maintain the deception that he was a hospital doctor. . . . There was good evidence that he also used deception in his personal relationships. In one relationship he claimed that he was a stockbroker and with another he claimed to be a member of the aristocracy. He cohabited with one woman for about two months, during which time he claimed that his mother was a judge and his father was a gangster. (pp. 199–200)

In other cases, the liars even demonstrate an awareness of why they tell their self-aggrandizing lies:

He claims he finds no satisfaction in how he really is, so has to "present a super image" and must never be a "bit player" but always "the centre of the stage." He has during his frequent sojourns in prison caused great problems for the authorities by his ability to create complex and difficult situations which have not infrequently led to official enquiries. He has managed to involve members of both Houses of Parliament and a myriad of officials from London to Strassbourg in these events. (Powell et al., 1983, p. 142)

HEROISM AND VICTIMIZATION THEMES

Treanor's (2012) analysis also found that in the majority of case studies (53%) the themes of the lies centered on heroism or victimization. Examples in the case report literature are easily found. Healy and Healy (1915) presented numerous cases of men and women whose lies cast them as the hero or heroine. For example, here are two cases:

Two years prior to the time we knew Marie she had worked up a story of adventure in which she was the heroine. She used the telephone to call for help, stating that she stood with a revolver covering a burglar. From this incident she gained a good deal of notoriety. The police found there was nothing to the case and later Marie herself made a confession. (pp. 96–97)

In the second case:

> The dramatic nature of his later stories seemed to fulfill the need which the boy felt of his being something which he was not, and very likely belonged to the same category of behavior he displayed when he attempted to impersonate a policeman in the middle of the night, and to pose as an amateur detective by telling stories of alleged exploits to newspaper reporters. A long story which he related even to us, involving his discovery of a suspicious man with a satchel and his use of a taxicab in search for him, was made up on the basis of his playing the part of a great man, a hero. (p. 139)

In other cases such as the following, the liars portray themselves in the victim role:

> A 26-year old Caucasian female, single mother, and nursing professional filed a complaint at a police station against unknown individuals on a Friday morning, after supposedly been robbed an hour before. She reported that she was on her daily way to work, as two unknown men crossed her course and asked for a cigarette lighter. At that moment, one of the men grabbed her unexpectedly from behind and held her in place while the other one kicked against her right thigh and knee. The woman resumed that she fell on the ground with her right side, whereupon one of the men strangled her ambidextrously to keep her to the ground. Furthermore, both men punched and kicked her against the head, face and body. In the end, they stole cash money and desisted from her. . . . Objective symptoms consisted of numerous diffuse, red, violet and blue skin discolorations of the face; in particular, at both cheeks and nose with a focus on the left side, ears, frontal and lateral sides of the neck, lateral sides of the torso, and the lateral area of the right thigh and knee (Fig. 1a–d). The discolorations appeared as fresh bruises. . . . Yet, because of a noticeably pasty skin appearance on the neck, resembling normal makeup, and for a proper assessment, the forensic expert removed makeup of the pertained regions of the body with white cotton pads. As a surprising result, all skin discolorations could be eliminated (Fig. 2a–d) and red, blue, green and

yellow paint adhered to the cotton wool (Fig. 3a–c). Therefore, the so-called "injuries" proved to be made up by paint. Further police investigations disclosed frequent reports against unknown persons, filed in the past by the woman. Ultimately, indications for a third-party interference did not exist. (Mauf et al., 2015, p. 33)

PURPOSE OF THE LIES

When one examines the various ways pathological lying has been described in the literature, one can see that the purposeless nature of the lies seems key to some researchers. However, the rationale for the lies is not critical to others' understanding of pathological lying. In the case study literature, one can find ample examples of individuals whose lies defy logic and seem to have no obvious function. For instance,

> During all our acquaintance with Adolf we have known his word to be absolutely untrustworthy. Many times he has descended upon his friends with quite unnecessary stories, leading to nothing but a lowering of their opinion of him. Repeatedly his concoctions have been without ascertainable purpose. (Healy & Healy, 1915, p. 159)

However, the inability to identify an external incentive for lying does not reasonably mean that the lies are told for no reason at all. There are certainly internal psychological motivations hidden from other's perceptions that drive much behavior. For instance, Ford et al. (1988) suggested that self-esteem needs may drive people to lie. In a number of cases, the authors opine that self-esteem needs may be driving the lying. For instance:

> First, it is clear that her lying was never initiated for any of the most common external motives. Her lies were not altruistic, white lies, and she did not lie to obtain money, sex, or a higher title (power) in her external environment. (She may have lied to enhance her social esteem or to feel power at being able to dupe another.) . . . Overall, it seemed clear from interviews that Lorraine's lying was strongly

driven by internal needs such as the need for excitement, attention, and enhanced self-esteem. (Birch et al., 2006, pp. 312–313)

Additionally, a number of case studies describe pathological liars who seem to have obviously clear reasons for lying:

> Mr. S first came into conflict with the law in his late teens. Since that time he has had over 100 convictions recorded against him involving theft and deception. He typically sets himself up with a false identity and persona and on the basis of cheque and credit card frauds supports himself in high style with fast cars the smartest of clothes and accommodation to match his pretensions. He is inevitably rapidly apprehended. It is clear from his own account and the evidence of his behaviour that the motivation is more that of being seen and accepted as a man of power and influence than to simply acquire goods and money. He is, as a result, an effective swindle but an ineffective criminal for he fails to take even the most minimal precautions against subsequent detection. Mr. S. consistently since early teens has substituted complex fantasies for the more solid achievements of reality. (Powell et al., 1983, p. 142)

IMPULSIVITY

Related to the idea that many pathological lies are purposeless, some have suggested that pathological liars lie impulsively, and so their actions may represent a form of dyscontrol that leads to their excesses (Hardie & Reed, 1998; Healy & Healy, 1915; B. H. King & Ford, 1988). There are case studies that mention impulsivity around the lies. For example,

> The patient noted that the lying has an impulsive quality about it; he often does not recognize that he has produced a falsehood until he "hears the words slipping out of [his] mouth." Then, largely out of shame and guilt and with recognition that he has lied, he embellishes the initial falsehood to avoid being discovered in the lie or being considered a fraud. (Modell et al., 1992, p. 443)

However, our review of the case studies aligns with Treanor's (2012) conclusion that impulsivity is seldom mentioned in descriptions of pathological liar cases. Thus, arguments that most pathological liars are suffering from impulsivity problems are not warranted based on the totality of available case reports.

COMPULSIVITY

Impulsivity refers to the tendency to act rashly or prematurely without any due consideration of one's actions, whereas *compulsivity* is the tendency to engage in repetitive behaviors, typically with no obvious purpose—and often with undesirable consequences. A review of the literature suggests that compulsivity may be a feature of pathological lying. After all, the term compulsive lying has historically been used synonymously with pathological lying (see Treanor, 2012). According to Figee et al. (2016),

> Compulsive behaviors are driven by repetitive urges and typically involve the experience of limited voluntary control over these urges, a diminished ability to delay or inhibit these behaviors, and a tendency to perform repetitive acts in a habitual or stereotyped manner. (p. 856)

B. H. King and Ford (1988) argued that the lying exhibited by pathological liars is often compulsive. Dike (2008) and Ford et al. (1988) also suggested that pathological lying may be compulsive. However, Treanor's (2012) review of historical case studies found compulsivity mentioned in only a small minority of cases (16%), suggesting that evidence of compulsive lying is uncommon in the case literature. In our analysis of case studies, we did find several examples in which compulsivity was mentioned. For example, Korkeila et al. (1995) reported this about two of their cases: "In both of our cases the symptoms involved a conspicuous compulsivity; deliberate as their stories were, their uncontrollability was evident" (p. 370). Healy and Healy (1915) described some of the liars they evaluated this way: "On closer inspection we find that the liar is no longer free, he has ceased to be master of his own lies, the lie has won" (p. 19). Thus, there is some evidence of compulsivity in the case literature but perhaps not as much as we had expected.

FACTITIOUS DISORDER AND PATHOLOGICAL LYING

A great number of the case reports of pathological liars involve deceptive patterns that could be construed as evidence of factitious disorder. As Dike (2020) argued, it is difficult to disentangle other disorders that involve frequent lying such as factitious disorder or Munchausen syndrome from pathological lying. He pointed to a case in which the lines between factitious disorder were quite blurred. In that case, a woman had clear indications of factitious disorder:

> Over a period of four years, she had caused her second daughter (third child), born prematurely, to be subjected to multiple surgical and medical interventions from which she almost died. She caused the child to have a surgically inserted gastrotomy tube for feeding as treatment for a reported swallowing dysfunction, injected pathogens she stole from her lab to cause her daughter grave illnesses, altered her daughter's sweat tests leading to a diagnosis of cystic fibrosis, and drained her blood causing severe anemia. Her daughter went into life-threatening anaphylactic shock during infusion of iron dextran for her anemia. In all, her daughter received 30 to 40 surgical and medical interventions in the four-year span. . . . In 2001, she informed her family that she [the mother] had just been diagnosed with bone cancer. (Dike, 2020, p. 433)

The woman went on to also claim that she had lost her hearing and required cochlear implants. She also reported that she was pregnant with twins. All of the maladies of her and her children were fabrications, clearly indicating factitious disorder. However, the woman also lied prolifically about other matters. For instance:

> She had a longstanding history of frequent lying behavior for no apparent reason. Right after her marriage in December 1998, she

told her husband she was taking classes for her PhD. She left home for classes on Tuesday and Thursday nights for one year, after which she announced that she had obtained her PhD. Her husband was surprised she could accomplish that feat in one year despite doing it part-time, but he was proud of her accomplishment. He reported that she had printed PhD on everything, including business cards and in her email address. (Dike, 2020, p. 433)

The woman also went on to get large tattoos in honor of twins she lost during pregnancy, although the pregnancy was also a lie. Dike's (2020) argument that pathological lying may be the superordinate category fits well with this case.

In another case, Pitt and Pitt (1984) described a case of factitious disorder in which a man was repeatedly seeking medical attention for heart attacks that he was not actually having, but also told lies unrelated or only tangentially related to the health concerns:

The patient stated that he was a nuclear physicist with the Nuclear Regulatory Commission and while investigating the Three-Mile Island nuclear accident had been exposed to a massive dose of radiation. . . . After discharge from the National Institutes of Health, he noted weight loss and anorexia but had not had any chest discomfort until the day of admission, when while investigating a "nuclear spill" in Michigan, he noted the occurrence of severe precordial chest pain. . . . The patient was noted to be evasive and doubts arose as to the veracity of his past history. The Nuclear Regulatory Commission was contacted and sent an investigator who determined that the patient was not a nuclear physicist and had not been associated with the agency. The patient was found to have had several previous hospitalizations for precordial chest pain. (pp. 137–138)

On the basis of the cases we have reviewed, we concur with Dike's (2020) position that pathological lying should be viewed as a broad category to which factitious disorder and other lying-related pathologies may belong.

ACCUSATORY PATHOLOGICAL LIARS

In some rare cases, the pathological liar tells lies that are accusatory in focus. For instance, Birch and colleagues (2006) presented the case of a 22-year-old woman named Lorraine who serially accused others of committing crimes against her:

> Lorraine's first major accusation occurred when she reported to the police receiving numerous menacing death threats over the telephone and in a letter from Vera, one of her female co-workers. Allegedly, Vera wanted Lorraine dead because she felt Lorraine was "interfering" in her relationship with her boyfriend. The content of the letter Lorraine submitted to police was graphic and dramatic: "You will die choking on your own blood. You are a walking image of death." As a result of Lorraine's allegations during this first incident, Vera was arrested and released with a notice to appear in court, and conditions to avoid all contact with Lorraine. Lorraine, however, eventually terminated her complaint when police became suspicious of the postmark on the letter, and requested that Lorraine submit to a polygraph test. (pp. 308–309)

Years later during a forensic examination, she confessed that she had concocted the story about Vera. When she was subsequently asked for the reason why she singled out Vera as the target of her false accusations, she stated, "Nothing. I don't have anything against Vera. Vera is a nice girl." Lorraine's accusatory lying did not end with Vera:

> About a year after this first major accusation, Lorraine made reports to police that Abby, her best friend since early grade school, had begun stalking her and, as in the case of Vera, had made numerous death threats over the telephone and in letters sent to Lorraine. Allegedly, Abby had suddenly developed a lesbian attraction to Lorraine and had become enraged when Lorraine did not reciprocate the romantic feelings. The threats were again very dramatic (e.g., "If I can't have you no one will"), and the letters Lorraine submitted to police contained threatening items that Abby had allegedly enclosed (e.g., a stolen and cut-up pair of Lorraine's underpants, as well as photographs taken of

Lorraine that were punctured around her neck). (Birch et al., 2006, p. 309)

Adding to the accusations, Lorraine later falsely accused Abby of abducting her at knife-point with the intent to kill her. Abby was arrested and criminally charged. Lorraine testified against her in court.

Not long after the supposed abduction, Lorraine accused her fiancé's ex-wife of sending death threats to her by mail and phone. According to Lorraine, the ex-wife wanted her dead because she had stolen her husband. Lorraine further accused the ex-wife of being involved in the previously discussed kidnapping attempt. The police arrested and charged the ex-wife because of the accusations. Immediately on the heels of the ex-wife's arrest, Lorraine started one fire that severely damaged her own mother's apartment. The next day she started a second fire that destroyed her own apartment. In both cases, she accused her fiancé's 3-year-old son of starting the fires. The child readily confessed when questioned.

Law enforcement officers finally realized that all of Lorraine's accusations were lies. When questioned about why she had told the lies, she offered, "I don't know why I did it. It was stupid. It was just one thing that happened at work. I just got carried away." On the basis of their extensive analysis of the case, Birch et al. (2006) concluded that Lorraine's accusatory lies were predominantly driven by internal needs rather than any discernable external gains. They noted that her lies were tied to her desire for attention, sympathy, emotional closeness from family and friends, and excitement. Although accusatory lies may be a somewhat rare form of pathological lying, the risk of substantial harm to others raises their importance in our opinions.

DISTRESS AND IMPAIRED FUNCTIONING

Most of the case studies of pathological liars suggest that lying leads to significant social, legal, and occupational problems, often causing great distress for the liar. For example:

Mr A was desperate. He was about to lose yet another job, not because he was at risk for being fired, but because his lying behavior had finally boxed him into a corner. He had lied repeatedly to his colleagues, telling them that he had an incurable disease and was receiving palliative treatment. Initially, his coworkers treated him with sensitivity and concern, but as the weeks wore on, the scrutiny of his colleagues became increasingly pointed. He had to tell more and more outrageous lies to cover his tracks and justify having a terminal illness. Finally, when the heat became too unbearable, he suddenly stopped going to work. On the face of it, it would seem Mr A told these lies to gain the sympathy of his colleagues, but the consequences of his lying, in terms of emotional distress and potential loss of job, far outweighed any perceived gain. Mr A had lost several other jobs in the past because of his lying, and he was becoming frustrated. Family members reported that he often told blatant lies, and even when confronted, and proved wrong, he still swore they were true. Mr A finally sought psychiatric help after concluding that he could not stop himself from lying. (Dike, 2008, p. 67)

In a case reported by Petra Garlipp (2017), a 32-year-old male engineer seemed to recognize the problems his lying was creating and seemed motivated to change:

He had noticed that he was very talented in constructing lies and that people believed him. The latest lie had been one he had told his family members, friends, and doctors. Specifically, he told them that he was suffering from a brain tumor. They believed him at first. He noted that he could skillfully manipulate others by lying, but in the end more conflict would result. His stated desire was to stop lying. . . . Interestingly enough, during day hospital treatment the patient regularly reported unusual events with a certain "sensation-seeking" quality. For example, he told other patients that he had rescued a former fellow patient from a criminal gang. (p. 320)

In another case from Modell and colleagues (1992), the patient seemed keenly aware of the significant dysfunctional effects of his lying. That distress led the patient to seek treatment:

The patient voluntarily sought treatment following a threat of divorce by his wife because of his frequent deceptions. Additionally, he admitted that his lying has been responsible for multiple job losses. He noted that he is very motivated to get help, fearing that the lying will continue to "ruin [his] life" if not stopped. (p. 443)

It is apparent in many of the pathological lying case studies, especially the ones for which there is extensive reporting from the subjects, that lying causes many negative consequences for the individuals and leads to marked distress.

The case studies exploring pathological liars span 130 years. During that time, the definitions of pathological lying that have been offered shifted, and the nature of the cases reported have varied in key ways. However, taking that body of case studies as a whole, one can discern common themes that are represented in the majority of cases. Advocates of different positions may point to particular cases to bolster their definitions and conceptualization of pathological lying, but we believe it is prudent to embrace a definition that can coherently address the largest number of cases. Our review suggests several features that are prevalent enough to be treated as key elements of pathological lying. Although some cases may lack one or more of these features, most seem to present several of them.

The majority of pathological lying cases describe individuals who frequently tell lies that are within the realm of possibility. They tell the lies chronically, often for years, and often beginning in childhood or early adulthood. They seem to be aware of the fact that they are lying, and while some cases may indicate impulsivity, it does not appear to be a key feature. Although some have suggested that the lies are purposeless, our review suggests that there are often indications of internal psychological motivations; these are merely inferred by observers, however, and it is not always clear that a liar is aware of their internal motivations. There are also some cases in which there seem to be external motivations for the lies. In the cases studies, the lies are often self-aggrandizing but also frequently place the liar in a victim role. The lies also tend to cause substantial impaired functioning and distress for the liars. Although somewhat limited in number, we believe that the accumulated case studies offer ample evidence against which the various definitions and explanations of pathological liars may be evaluated.

5

Pathological Aspects of Lying

The distinction between normal and abnormal, or healthy functioning and psychopathology, has been controversial. Some scholars, writers, and clinicians have long recognized differences between normal and pathological functioning, whereas others have suggested that there is no distinction at all. The debate tends to center on concerns of correctly identifying clusters of symptoms that typically occur together, usually to inform a treatment, versus believing that labels are artificially created and may lead to stigma and other negative consequences. It is worth noting that this debate appears to be found only within the mental health professions (e.g., psychiatry and psychology), as there is not much controversy about whether the biological study of pathology or pathophysiology is real or artificially created to stigmatize others.

The terms *pathology* and *pathological* come from the Greek words *pathos* and *logos*. Logos (λόγς) means "word" or "reason" and is often part of a word describing an area of study (e.g., psycho*logy*, bio*logy*); pathos

https://doi.org/10.1037/0000305-005
Pathological Lying: Theory, Research, and Practice, by D. A. Curtis and C. L. Hart

(πάθος) means "suffering," "experience," or "emotion." Pathos can be found in several English words, such as pathetic, empathy, sympathy, apathy, sociopath, and psychopath (Merriam-Webster, 2021). Pathology would be roughly translated as the study of suffering, and within medicine it has tended to be understood as the study of diseases (Merriam-Webster, 2021). Adding the prefix of psych to pathology, yielding psychopathology, would be understood as the study of suffering of the soul or study of mental suffering and disorders.

The German psychologist Hermann Ebbinghaus (1908) stated that "psychology has a long past, yet its real history is short" (p. 3). Similarly, psychopathology has a long past but a short history. "Since there has been human, abnormality has been found" (Curtis & Kelley, 2020a, p. 16). People have sought to understand and explain abnormal behaviors since early recorded history, but the formal study of psychopathology is more recent. Evidence of psychological interventions can be found from early recorded history (Benjamin & Baker, 2004). Treatments of psychopathology have included natural and supernatural methods. Such techniques can be found in trephining individuals (by drilling a hole in a person's skull to release spirits from a person's head), shamanic practices of dancing and singing, balancing bodily humors (increasing or decreasing bodily fluids), examining the structure of a person's head (referred to as phrenology), exorcism, prayer, medicine, and talk therapy (Benjamin & Baker, 2004; Curtis & Kelley, 2020a; Frances, 2013; C. G. Gross, 1999). However, nosology (science of classifying diseases) and the formal study of psychopathology were not present before the 1900s (Blashfield et al., 2014; Jaspers, 1913/1963).

To fully understand pathological aspects of lying, or pathological lying, classification systems are discussed in this chapter. Additionally, how these systems function to differentiate normality from psychopathology are examined. Classification systems are foundational to build on as we draw from the previous chapters and the research on normative aspects of lying. We compare features of normative lying to pathological aspects of lying by highlighting nosological frameworks and using a model of psycho-pathology. Subsequently, we present research findings that distinguish pathological lying from prolific lying and normative lying. Last, we discuss other features of pathological lying.

CLASSIFICATION AND NOSOLOGY

Classification is a central trait of humans. Blashfield and Burgess (2007) made the strong case that "just as water is basic to human existence, classification is fundamental to human cognition" (p. 113). When kids begin to speak, they may call every four-legged hairy creature a "dog." Dogs, cats, horses, bunnies, squirrels—all are categorized as dogs. As language develops and broadens, people are able to discriminate categorically, making classifications and distinctions. Classification serves several functions. Consider the image of a dog. When asking several people to think of a dog, various images may come to mind. For example, people may conjure the image of a black and white dalmatian, a big hairy German shepherd, a small terrier, a sleek Doberman pinscher, or a playful boxer. Thinking of each of these words draws more specific imagery than the general label of dog. Classification allows a mental representation. The more specific the classifications system is, the more specificity of language and thought.

It can be argued that the formal study of psychopathology can be attributed to Philippe Pinel (1801, 1813). In 1801, Pinel published a classification system of mental disorders. He discussed four major categories: melancholias, manias with delirium, manias without delirium, and dementia or mental deterioration. This early work of Pinel largely influenced classification systems that emerged more than a century later. Others credit the formal recognition of psychopathology as an area of study to Karl Jaspers (1913/1963), who published a comprehensive book titled *Allgemeine Psychopathologie* (General Psychopathology). Around the same time, Emil Kraepelin (1919), following in the footsteps of Pinel, established nomenclature for two broad classifications.

The early work of these scholars, physicians, and psychiatrists to establish classification systems was prompted by recognizing, discussing, describing, and promoting understanding into the areas of psychopathology that were observed within the world, primarily from practitioners. Similar to any classification system, such as biological taxonomy (domain, kingdom, phylum, class, order, family, genus, species), psychiatry and psychology was seeking to organize mental disorders to achieve the goals of classification systems. Blashfield and Burgess (2007) suggested six goals of classification: (a) nomenclature, (b) information retrieval, (c) description, (d) prediction, (e) concept formation, and (f) sociopolitical. Thus, classification promotes language of a construct, phenomenon, object, or species and adds to cognitive complexity in thinking about the category.

Classification is inescapable. Consider the broad construct of psychopathology. A number of people believe there exists a distinction between normative behavior and behavior that can be pathological. On the other hand, some people may believe that there is no such thing as normal or that everyone has their own, relative, normal. Both groups have classified human behavior, the former making a distinction and the latter classifying all behavior as normal. It is the method by which classification is used and whether there is an established nomenclature with consensus that tends to elicit controversy.

In debates about classification methods, advocates can generally be divided into *lumpers* and *splitters*. The difference between lumpers and splitters was found in the early work of in the classification of mammals, where the lumpers have an inclination to group more broadly and emphasize similarities while splitters have the propensity to seek out more specific characteristics that are distinguishable (Simpson, 1945). Psychology has witnessed long-standing debates between lumpers and splitters, specifically regarding organization of the discipline or the structure of the divisions (Dewsbury, 1997). The debate has even been evidenced within psychiatry, where authors have discussed the benefits and drawbacks of each approach for diagnostic categories (e.g., Leventhal, 2012; Mandy et al., 2012).

There are good arguments posed for each perspective as well as potential biases and drawbacks. Broad categorizations highlight similarities and homogeneity and may offer an ease of use or recall (less information). The drawback of lumping is that it may overgeneralize or not recognize differences that are subtle and distinguishing. Using the dog analogy, if every dog were given the general label of dog, then there would be a difficulty with communication when referencing a specific dog (e.g., terrier or German shepherd). Thus, splitting allows for more specificity of characteristics within categories and facilitates more precision in communication. However, there is a limit to splitting. At what point does splitting various elements of a dog make it so unique that its characteristics do not seem to be a part of any broader category? There are advantages and disadvantages to using either lumper or splitter approaches, but each level of analysis offers utility and works with the other.

The public may have two basic classifications for all psychopathology: crazy or normal. The judicial system has used two broad classification categories: sanity or insanity. Recall that the early pioneers, Pinel and Kraepelin, had few basic categories for classification. Before the publication of the first edition of the *Diagnostic and Statistical Manual of Mental Disorders* (*DSM-I*; American Psychiatric Association, 1952), Thomas Moore conducted a factor analysis that resulted in eight factors of symptom groupings (Blashfield et al., 2014). The original *DSM-I* consisted of 128 diagnostic categories and 132 pages, whereas the *DSM-5* originally had a total of 541 diagnostic categories that was trimmed down to 151 diagnostic categories and 947 pages (Blashfield et al., 2014). In contrast, the 11th edition of the *International Statistical Classification of Diseases and Related Health Problems* (*ICD-11*; World Health Organization [WHO], 2019) has "17,000 diagnostic categories, with over 100,000 medical diagnostic index terms," although psychological disorders constitute only a portion of these (WHO, 2021b, para. 3).

What conclusion can be drawn from such information? Some may postulate that the increase in diagnostic categories is out of control. Are practitioners haphazardly producing numerous labels to pathologize the world? Is big pharma seeking to crank out new pathologies to gain monetarily for mass production of medicine? Allen Frances (2013), former chair of the *DSM-IV* Task Force, criticized the changes in the *DSM* and stated that there is a diagnostic inflation. Frances discussed his concerns about the pharmaceutical industry and psychiatric medications. On the other hand, the increase in diagnostic categories may represent diagnostic sophistication, or a recognition of phenomenon that may have been overlooked or broadly lumped into another classification. Subsequent chapters clarify how a lack of specificity in diagnostic categories can lead clinicians to provide a different diagnosis when they are confronted with symptoms and there is not a diagnostic category. Thus, psychopathological classification could be viewed as mirroring human cognitive development, in that language aids in cognitive complexity.

There is a real danger for clinicians, researchers, and even patients of mental health providers in avoiding nomenclature in classification. Take the patient who is suicidal and suffering from major depressive disorder. When the person hesitantly seeks out psychotherapy and confesses being in intense pain and wanting to end it all by suicide, classification and language are important for all parties. What would be the implications of telling the person that there is nothing wrong with them and that they are normal, not suffering from any psychopathology? Might the person accept this statement and become less suicidal and less depressed, or is it possible that the person would think that they are being dismissed? The consequences could be severe. Nomenclature also helps clinicians communicate precisely with each other. Further, knowing that what they experience has a name, others have experienced similar symptoms, and there is a possibility for treatment often instills hope in patients.

In previous chapters, we demonstrated how practitioners have historically interacted with people who have engaged in pathological lying. The clinicians have observed and experienced instances of the phenomenon. Some of them have even classified the phenomenon by providing nomenclature such as pseudologia phantastica or pathological lying. However, this nomenclature has mostly been picked up in smaller clinical circles and not by major nosological systems.

MAJOR NOSOLOGICAL SYSTEMS

Diagnosis is not a malevolent process aimed at assigning damning labels. On the contrary, diagnosis is a simple step in the part of a process to help others. A diagnosis is merely a label for a set of symptoms that typically cluster together. Nothing more, nothing less. So why, then, is are diagnoses or nosologies regarded as (or even taught to be) menacing entities? Most of the problems that arise from the classification of mental disorders emerge from society rather than from practitioners (Curtis & Kelley, 2020a).

Clinicians do not generate arbitrary labels to stigmatize others. Most practitioners, now and in the past, have sought terminology to fully understand, communicate, and to ultimately help those who were suffering.

"The field of psychopathology is no different . . . classification of mental disorders is the basis for organizing scientific knowledge in the field" (Blashfield & Burgess, 2007, p. 93). These systems of classification promote research of psychological disorders and foster a process for mental health professionals to aid in the treatment of individuals. For the practitioner, the nomenclature for a diagnosis has always been merely a label to understand and help. The historical process of health care professionals has always been a process of assessing, making a diagnosis, and providing a treatment:

Assessment → Diagnosis → Treatment

Major nosological systems have focused on nomenclature, discussing the classifications of a variety of psychological disorders. While the American Psychiatric Association published its first statistical classification in 1844, the *DSM-I* was originally published in 1952 (American Psychiatric Association, 1952, 2013). The fifth and current edition, the *DSM-5*, was published in 2013 and has undergone significant changes to increase specificity and produce research markers for psychological disorders. The *DSM-5* defines mental disorder as

> A syndrome characterized by clinically significant disturbance in an individual's cognition, emotion regulation, or behavior that reflects a dysfunction in the psychological, biological, or developmental processes underlying mental functioning . . . associated with significant distress or disability in social, occupational, or other important activities. (American Psychiatric Association, 2013, p. 20)

Parallel to the *DSM*, the *ICD* is a broader nosology of diseases and health problems. Housed within the *ICD* are mental, behavioral, neurodevelopmental, and sleep–wake disorders. The *ICD-10* defined disorder as a "clinically recognizable set of symptoms or behaviour associated in most cases with distress and with interference with personal functions" (WHO, 1992, p. 11).

THEORY OF PATHOLOGICAL LYING

Aligning with the frameworks of psychopathology found within the major nosological systems, Curtis and Kelley (2016, 2020a) suggested a model to help discern abnormal from normal. They suggested the use of the four Fs: frequency, function, feeling pain, and fatal (Curtis & Kelley, 2020a; see Figure 5.1). The four Fs were proposed as an adaptation of Nolen-Hoeksema's (2007, 2011) four Ds (deviance, dysfunction, distress, danger) and suggested to better map onto the major nosological systems (Curtis & Kelley, 2020a). For example, deviance mostly described the small percentage of individuals who exhibit psychopathology, whereas frequency more precisely described psychopathology in terms of the increase or decrease in a behavior, the duration of the behavior, and the small percentage of individuals who display similar patterns. The four Fs are a model to examine psychological disorders, revealing that a behavioral excess or deficiency that occurs for some duration within a smaller group of the population and often causes significant impairment in functioning, distress, and poses risks to the individual or others. An example can be found in examining major depressive disorder. Most people have experienced sadness or even had a depressive mood. However, a smaller group of people

The Four Fs of Abnormality

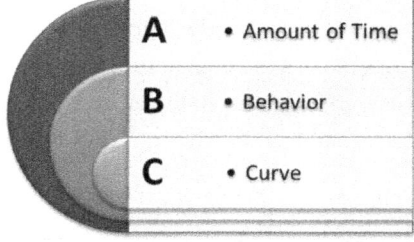

1. Frequency
2. Function
3. Feeling Pain
4. Fatal

A • Amount of Time

B • Behavior

C • Curve

Figure 5.1

From *Abnormal Psychology: Myths of "Crazy"* (3rd ed., p. 10), by D. A. Curtis and L. Kelley, 2020, Kendall Hunt. Copyright 2020 by Kendall Hunt Publishing Company. Reprinted with permission.

(approximately 7%) exhibit at least five of nine symptoms for at least 2 weeks that significantly impairs their functioning (not going to work, not getting out of bed), brings about pain, and may be fatal (suicide risks).

Curtis (2019) suggested the use of this model as a theoretical framework for understanding pathological lying. The theoretical application emerged following the publication of the frequency data on lying from Serota and colleagues (2010; Serota & Levine, 2015). Their important findings on lie frequency revealed that although the average number of lies told per day is around two, the distribution of lying behavior is positively skewed (see Figure 5.2).

The positive skew indicates that most people do not lie often and the majority of lies told per day are told by a smaller group of individuals. Serota and colleagues (2010) referred to the smaller group of people who told excessive lies as *prolific liars*. Drawing from the four Fs, it was reasoned that pathological liars may be a subset of the group of people who told an excessive amount of lies per day. Specifically, within the group of people who tell an excessive number of lies per day, there may be some whose lies cause impaired functioning and feeling pain and could be fatal. This theoretical framework was used in a study that we conducted and describe in the next section, which discusses the research on pathological lying.

PATHOLOGICAL LYING RESEARCH

In the previous chapter, we presented several cases of pathological lying. Case studies are a crucial component of the science and practice of psychotherapy (Davison & Lazarus, 2007). Cases studies are useful and arguably an important first step in research because they reveal observations of a phenomenon. Often, clinical findings fuel laboratory studies. This is certainly the case with pathological lying, in that numerous case studies documented the existence of pathological lying as it occurred within clinical contexts. There should exist "a two-way street" between the laboratory and the clinic, each contributing to the other (Davison & Lazarus, 2007). However, many of the case studies and much of the documentation on pathological lying have resided at the clinic address. There has been less

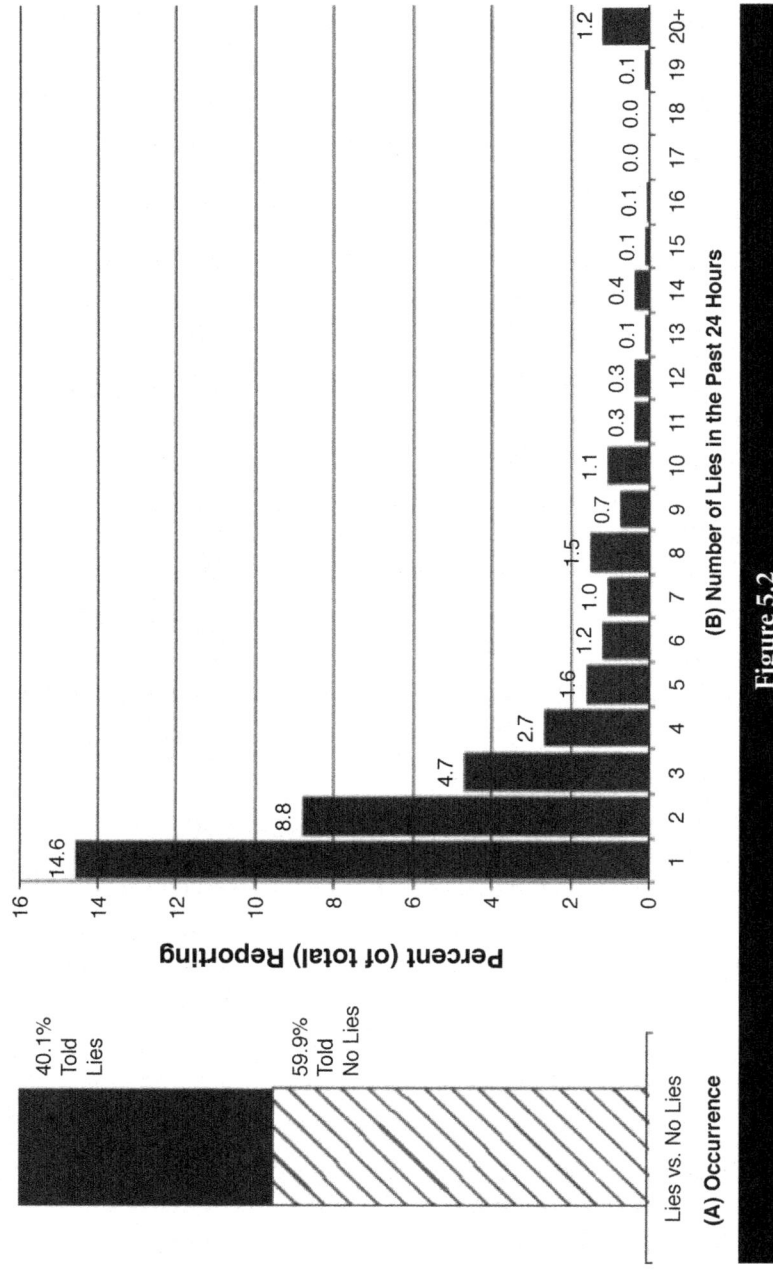

Figure 5.2

Distribution of lies told per day. From "The Prevalence of Lying in America: Three Studies of Self-Reported Lies," by K. B. Serota, T. R. Levine, and F. J. Boster, 2010, *Human Communication Research, 36*(1), p. 9 (https://doi.org/10.1111/j.1468-2958.2009.01366.x). Copyright 2010 by Oxford University Press. Reprinted with permission.

traffic from researchers studying pathological lying. Having discussed various case studies, we now turn our attention to some of the research findings from the scarce empirical investigations of pathological lying. We also discuss the few studies that have analyzed larger samples of pathological lying.

One of the earliest documented studies of pathological lying was conducted by Healy and Healy in 1915. Along with presenting case studies, they reported an analysis of 1,000 young repeat offenders (694 males, 306 females, ranging in age from 6 to 22 years). They examined the number of offenders in which lying was "a notable and excessive trait," finding that it was counted in 15% of males and 26% of females (p. 5). However, Healy and Healy stated that "the exact number of pathological liars is not determinable" in their analyses but assumed it to be "8 to 10 of the 1000" (p. 5).

In 1933, Wiersma sought to analyze common features of 30 patients who presented with pseudologia fantastica. He used the data of these patients' histories to conclude that those with pseudologia fantastica were lazy, not industrious, were highly emotional, often changed professions, and were vain. Wiersma also suggested that the pathological liars possessed characteristics similar of a nervous temperament.

About 50 years later, B. H. King and Ford (1988) revisited pathological lying by reviewing 72 cases of pseudologia fantastica found within 26 reports beginning in 1891. B. H. King and Ford's analysis indicated that pathological lying was equally represented among men and women, had a typical onset in adolescence, the subjects' intelligence was average to above average, and half of the reports involved some engagement in crime. B. H. King and Ford also reported on the incidence of central nervous system abnormality, finding that 40% of the cases demonstrated some central nervous system abnormality (see Table 5.1).

Within the vein of neuroscience, Modell et al. (1992) examined a case of pathological lying through brain scanning technology. They used single-photon emission computed tomography (SPECT) of the brain of a 35-year-old man who identified as a pathological liar. The man indicated that his lying behaviors impaired his relational and occupational functioning. He sought treatment after his wife threatened divorce because of

Table 5.1

Analysis of CNS Abnormality Among Patients With Pseudologia Fantastica

	Male ($n = 35$) %	Female ($n = 32$) %	All ($N = 67$) %
Epilepsy	26	3	15
Abnormal EEG	11	3	7
Head trauma	9	6	7
CNS infection	6	9	7
Congenital abnormalities	3	6	4
Anoxia	3	3	3
Syncope	0	6	3
Other	3	3	3
All	43	34	39

Note. CNS = central nervous system; EEG = electroencephalogram. From "Pseudologia Fantastica," by B. H. King and C. V. Ford, 1988, *Acta Psychiatrica Scandinavica, 77*(1), p. 3 (https://doi.org/10.1111/j.1600-0447.1988.tb05068.x). Copyright 1988 by John Wiley & Sons, Inc. Reprinted with permission.

his excessive lies. The patient reported that his lies were often impulsive, and then he subsequently experienced shame and guilt. He also indicated that his lies tended to be embellished to maintain an initial lie. They found that the patient had a normal physical examination and tested negative for drugs of abuse. Modell and colleagues discovered that the functional imaging scans indicated an abnormally low tracer uptake in the right hemithalamus (see Figure 5.3). They suggested that the decrease in the tracer uptake in the right hemithalamus might be related to decreased blood flow and impairment in this brain region. From this, Modell and colleagues concluded, "We therefore believe that the decreased functional activity of the right hemithalamus of our patient (and the lesser decrease of the right inferior frontal cortex) may be responsible for his tendency to lie impulsively" (p. 446).

Continuing to explore brain imaging technologies and pathological lying, Yang and colleagues (2005) contributed a novel brain imaging study of deceitful individuals. They assessed 12 people who pathologically lied (classified as liars), 16 antisocial control subjects, and 21 normal controls

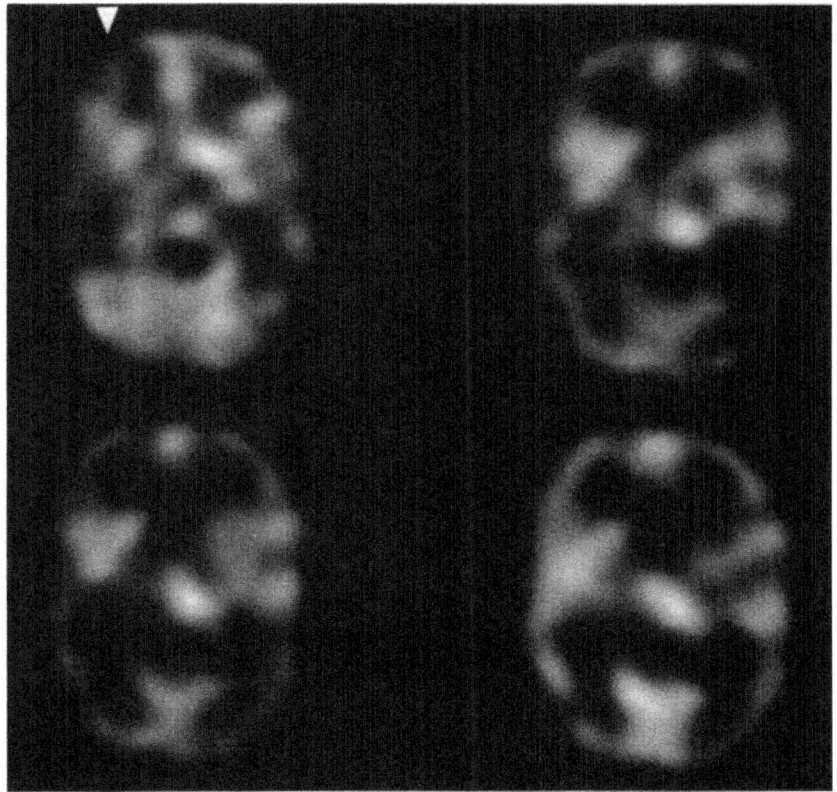

Figure 5.3

SPECT scan of a pathological lying case. The top left section is through the lower frontal lobes and shows the decrease in right inferior frontal cortical tracer uptake in regional cerebral blood flow (arrow) as compared with the normal uptake on the left. The top right and two bottom sections show sequential cuts through the thalamus; the marked decrease in tracer uptake by the right hemithalamus and the slightly elevated uptake by the left are apparent on these sections. SPECT = single-photon emission computed tomography. From "Pathological Lying Associated With Thalamic Dysfunction Demonstrated by [99mTc]HMPAO SPECT," by J. G. Modell, J. M. Mountz, and C. V. Ford, 1992, *The Journal of Neuropsychiatry and Clinical Neurosciences*, 4(4), p. 445 (https://doi.org/10.1176/jnp.4.4.442). Copyright 1992 by American Psychiatric Association Publishing. Reprinted with permission.

subjects. The liars were classified based on meeting four criteria: (a) pathological lying item from the Psychopathy Checklist—Revised (PCL-R; Hare, 1991), (b) conning/manipulative behavior on the PCL-R, (c) deceitfulness criterion for the *DSM-IV* (American Psychiatric Association, 1994), and (d) malingering based on whether they admitted to lying for obtaining sickness benefits during an interview (Yang et al., 2005). Results indicated that liars had a 22.2% increase in prefrontal white matter compared with normal control subjects and 25.7% increase compared with antisocial control subjects. Further, liars had showed a 14.2% decrease in prefrontal gray matter compared with the normal controls, though not statistically significant. The liar group had more prefrontal white matter than the control and antisocial groups (see Figure 5.4).

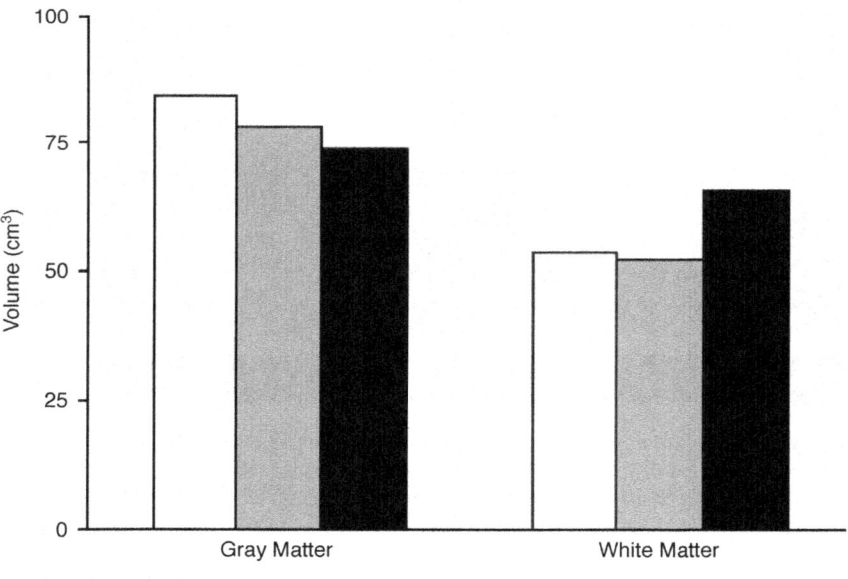

Figure 5.4

Prefrontal gray and white matter volumes in liars (black), normal controls (white), and antisocial controls (gray). From "Prefrontal White Matter in Pathological Liars," by Y. Yang, A. Raine, T. Lencz, S. Bihrle, L. Lacasse, and P. Colletti, 2005, *The British Journal of Psychiatry*, *187*(4), p. 322 (https://doi.org/10.1192/bjp.187.4.320). Copyright 2005 by Cambridge University Press. Reprinted with permission.

The authors discussed that one of the most significant findings of the study was that of the increase in prefrontal white matter and decrease in gray-to-white ratio for the liar group. Yang and colleagues (2005) contrasted this finding to children with autism, one feature of which is the propensity for honesty or lying less (Sodian, 1991; Sodian & Frith, 1992; Talwar & Lee, 2002b). Yang et al. (2005) suggested that the liars in their study revealed the converse pattern of gray-to-white ratios compared with children who have autism. Spence (2005), in an invited commentary, suggested that the increased prefrontal white matter may be a predisposition to lying, although it is not clear which comes first, brain structure or the lying. Spence went on to critique the classification of pathological lying because it was primarily used by Yang and colleagues (2005) with regard to antisocial lying and may not account for all aspects of pathological lying. Yang et al. (2005), recognizing the need for further investigation, suggested a working hypothesis "that increased prefrontal white matter developmentally provides the individual with the cognitive capacity to lie" (p. 323).

Following this study, Yang et al. (2007) published another study that examined the white matter in four prefrontal subregions: inferior frontal, middle frontal, orbitofrontal, and superior frontal cortices. The sample in that study included 10 people classified as liars, 20 normal controls, and 14 antisocial controls. The classification criteria were the same used in the previous study by Yang and colleagues (2005). Their results indicated that liars showed an increase in white matter in the inferior cortex (32%–36% increase), middle cortex (28%–32% increase), and orbitofrontal cortex (22%–26% increase). They found no significant differences for gray matter across the four subregions (see Figure 5.5).

The researchers suggested that one possible explanation is that these prefrontal structures may play a role within pathological liars and their tendency to tell excessive. However, they discussed the possibility that pathological lying could result in changes in these brain structures. Yang and colleagues (2007) concluded by suggesting a future longitudinal study to assess pathological lying from childhood to adulthood to better address the concern of whether pathological lying is a result of the brain structure variation or whether lying results in this morphology. Although these

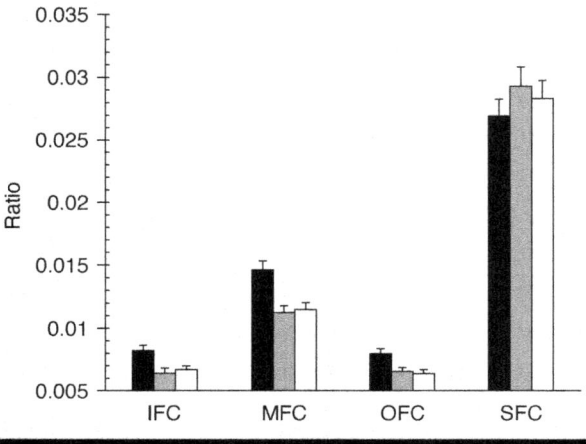

Figure 5.5

Whole-brain-corrected prefrontal white matter volumes in the inferior frontal cortex (IFC), middle frontal cortex (MFC), orbitofrontal cortex (OFC), and superior frontal cortex (SFC) in pathological liars (■), normal controls (□) and antisocial controls (▦). Vertical lines indicate the standard error of the mean. From "Localisation of Increased Prefrontal White Matter in Pathological Liars," by Y. Yang, A. Raine, K. L. Narr, T. Lencz, L. LaCasse, P. Colletti, and A. W. Toga, 2007, *The British Journal of Psychiatry, 190*(2), p. 5 (https://doi.org/10.1192/bjp.bp.106.025056). Copyright 2007 by Cambridge University Press. Reprinted with permission.

studies should be commended for initiating research in the area of neuroscience and pathological lying, there are several limitations and a need for more studies.

PATHOLOGICAL LYING: THEORETICAL AND EMPIRICAL SUPPORT FOR A DIAGNOSTIC ENTITY

More recently, we conducted a study to test whether the theoretical model of the four Fs of psychopathology could determine whether pathological lying was as a distinct group, separate from normative lying (Curtis & Hart, 2020b). We recruited 623 participants from various platforms: Facebook, Reddit/samplesize, Psych Forums, and a university. All participants were asked to complete the Survey of Pathological Lying (see Appendix A, this volume) or Survey of Lying Behaviors, Survey of Others' Pathological Lying, the Lying in Everyday Situations Scale (Hart et al.,

2019), the Distress Questionnaire—5 (DQ-5; Batterham et al., 2016), and a demographics questionnaire. We were specifically interested in examining whether pathological lying would meet the criteria of a disorder based on the *DSM-5* and *ICD-10* parameters as well as the standards of the four Fs. Essentially, we predicted that if pathological lying was a distinct disorder, then people who have expressed being a pathological liar would tell more lies than others for a longer duration, their lies would impair their functioning, they would experience more distress from their lies, and their lies would put them or others in danger more compared with nonpathological liars. Further, as Serota and colleagues (2010; Serota & Levine, 2015) discovered a statistical grouping of people who lied excessively that they referred to a group of prolific liars, we investigated whether pathological liars differed from this group. We predicted that pathological liars would be a group of people carved out of the prolific liar group, in that they would share features of telling excessive lies but would differ by having impaired functioning, feeling pain, and meeting the fatal criteria (see Figure 5.6). Thus, lying can be discussed by referencing three different groups: normative liars, prolific liars, and pathological liars.

In addition to testing the model of the four Fs, we sought to examine other aspects that have been referenced in literature. Because pathological lying has been referenced to consist of a compulsive–impulsive element, we examined whether pathological liars would indicate that their lying was not entirely in their control and that it provided relief from anxiety. We predicted that the pathological lying group would indicate that their lying had these features of compulsivity. Regarding the self-perception of motivation to tell lies, we asked participants whether they believed that they told lies for no specific reason. We predicted that pathological liars would more strongly endorse that item, claiming to tell lies without a specific goal or motivation.

THE HYDRA HYPOTHESIS

In Greek mythology, the Hydra (Λερναῖα Ὕδρα), was a mythical beast that was created to defeat Hercules. The Hydra had a unique feature: If its head was chopped off, three new heads would grow to replace it.

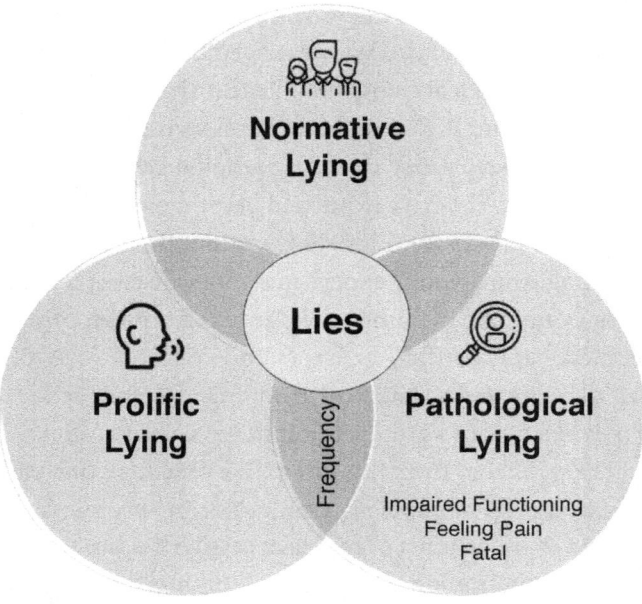

Figure 5.6

Classification distinctions of normative lying, prolific lying, and pathological lying.

Thus, the hydra was an unyielding mythological character. A large part of early psychological tradition (e.g., Freud, Jung) was to use mythos in psychological theory to understand or explain human processes.

Carrying the influence of Jung, J. Peterson (2017) discussed lying as a hydra, stating that lies have the propensity to grow in complexity. For example, children may tell one lie to avoid getting into trouble for some act, such as microwaving a fork or digging up the garden. Then, when interrogated by another parent or other siblings, the child may feel compelled to tell additional lies to maintain the plausibility of the first lie. We reasoned that the tendency to tell numerous lies from an initial lie, the Hydra hypothesis, would be a feature of pathological lying, in which excessive lies are told to maintain an initial lie. To explore this notion of pathological lying in which lies can become excessive and chronic, we asked participants if they believed their lies tend to grow from an initial lie.

We predicted that pathological liars would indicate that their lies grow from an initial lie more so than nonpathological liars.

RESULTS

To examine whether the fit of the frequency of lies aligned with self-identified pathological lying, we conducted a negative binomial regression due to it being more robust in handling overdispersed count or rate data (Gardner et al., 1995). In examining the model of lies told fitting with self-identified pathological lying, the likelihood ratio chi-square test indicated that the model was a significant improvement in fit and the classification was retained. Thus, the pathological lying group was supported. Participants were asked if they have been formally diagnosed (by a licensed mental health professional) with a psychological disorder. A frequency analysis revealed that 67% of the people in the pathological lying group reported that they had never been diagnosed with a psychological disorder.

The demographics of our sample consisted of adults aged 18 to 20 years with more female participants. Although the majority of participants were Caucasian (59%), other ethnicities were represented, including Hispanic and/or Latinx (25%), multiracial (8%), African American/Black (4%), Asian/Asian American/Pacific Islander (4%), Native American and/or Alaskan Native (2%). The participants ranged in education, and a majority indicated that their annual income was under $25,000 (85%). We found no significant differences between the pathological liar group and non-pathological liar group with regard to age, sex, education, income, and ethnicity. Thus, individuals in the pathological lying group did not represent a specific cultural group or reveal specific demographic factors that distinguished them from nonpathological liars.

Four Fs

Regarding the four Fs, we found support that pathological liars consisted of people who told excessive lies that impaired their functioning, brought about feeling pain, and was more fatal (dangerous to themselves or others). Regarding the frequency criteria, most people (87%) who engaged in pathological lying did so for longer than 6 months, they told an average of 10 lies per day, and made up approximately 8% to 13% of the sample. More than half (54%) of the pathologically lying participants reported that they had been telling numerous lies for longer than 5 years, with typical onset during childhood and adolescence (3–20 years), although most participants (62%) indicated the onset was in adolescence (see Table 5.2).

Regarding the number of lies told, there was a positively skewed distribution in which the most common response of pathological liars was that they reported telling one lie per day and a smaller group reported telling many more lies ($M = 9.99$, $SD = 11.17$, $Mdn = 7$, Mode = 1, $N = 82$, Max = 66 lies, 95% confidence interval [CI] [7.5, 12.44], skewness = 2.27, $SE = 0.27$, and kurtosis = 7.20, $SE = 0.53$; see Figure 5.7). Although the modal lie was one, the majority of participants who were pathological liars told five or more lies per day. Pathological liars reported telling more lies in a face-to-face context within friendships and social relationships. The fewest lies were reported being told to those seen occasionally in a written, phone, or internet format.

Individuals who engaged in pathological lying had greater impairment in functioning compared with nonpathological liars with regard to telling lies across areas of social relationships, occupational, financial, and

Table 5.2

Amount of Time Engaged in Pathological Lying, From Curtis and Hart (2020b)

Duration	Frequency	%
3 months	10	12.8
6 months	8	10.3
1 year	4	5.1
1–5 years	14	17.9
More than 5 years	42	53.8
Total	78	100.0

Note. Adapted from "Pathological Lying: Theoretical and Empirical Support for a Diagnostic Entity," by D. A. Curtis and C. L. Hart, 2020, *Psychiatric Research and Clinical Practice*, 2(2), p. 65 (https://doi.org/10.1176/appi.prcp.20190046). CC BY 4.0.

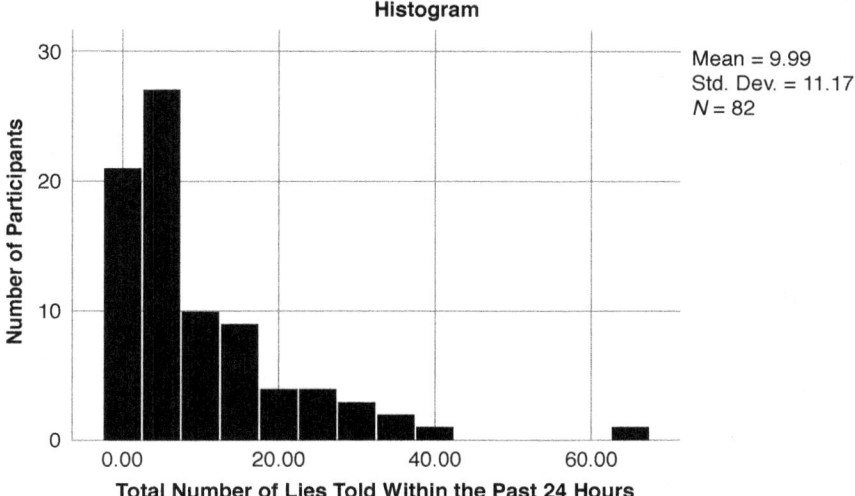

Figure 5.7

Distribution of pathological liars' lies told per day. Adapted from "Pathological Lying: Theoretical and Empirical Support for a Diagnostic Entity," by D. A. Curtis and C. L. Hart, 2020, *Psychiatric Research and Clinical Practice, 2*(2), pp. 62–69 (https://doi.org/10.1176/appi.prcp.20190046). CC BY 4.0.

legal contexts. However, the greatest area of impairment in functioning was found to be within the area of social relationships. Following relational problems, financial concerns were also indicated to be an area of concern for pathological liars. They indicated that legal contexts were an area of least impaired functioning.

The feeling pain criteria was met in two ways. First, individuals who engaged in pathological lying reported that their lying caused them significantly more distress compared with individuals who were in the nonpathological lying group. Additionally, individuals in the pathological lying group reported significantly more general psychological distress compared with those in the nonpathological lying group based on the DQ-5 (Batterham et al., 2016). In fact, by using the DQ-5 based on suggested cut points for sensitivity and specificity, we found that approximately 9% of the pathological lying group was identified based on sensitivity, and 8% of individuals met the cut point for specificity. Thus, researchers and clinicians may consider employing the DQ-5 as a tool to assist with assessing individuals as pathological liars, considering these cut points.

The fatal criterion was assessed by asking participants if their lying put themselves or others in danger. Our findings indicated that pathological liars reported that their lying led to more danger for themselves or others compared with individuals in the nonpathological lying group.

Cluster Analysis and the Four Fs

In addition to running other statistical analyses for testing the fitness of our model of identifying pathological liars, we conducted a k-means cluster analysis to determine whether pathological lying would represent a distinct group based on the Four Fs. Thus, we converted the frequency of lies, functioning, distress, and danger into Z-scores and then ran the cluster analysis. Two clusters were found from the analysis of the Four Fs: pathological lying and nonpathological lying (see Figure 5.8). An analysis of variance revealed statistical significance for functioning, $F(1, 513) = 533.80, p < .001$; distress,

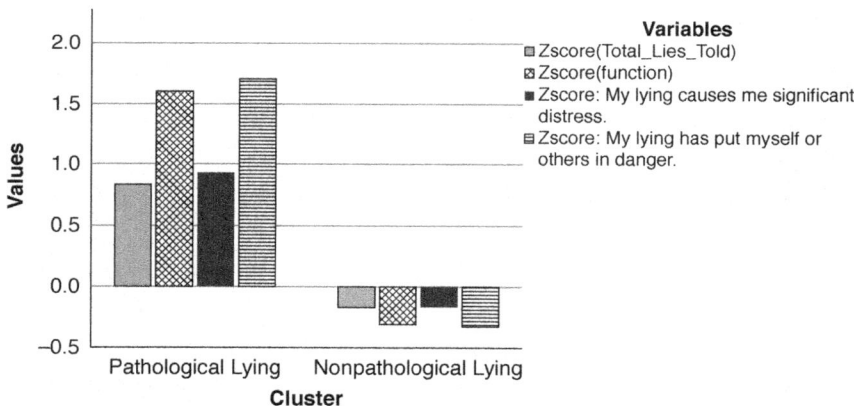

Figure 5.8

Cluster analysis of pathological and nonpathological lying. Adapted from "Pathological Lying: Theoretical and Empirical Support for a Diagnostic Entity," by D. A. Curtis and C. L. Hart, 2020, *Psychiatric Research and Clinical Practice, 2*(2), pp. 62–69 (https://doi.org/10.1176/appi.prcp.20190046). CC BY 4.0.

$F(1, 513) = 100.77, p < .001$; danger, $F(1, 513) = 650.21, p < .001$; and lie frequency, $F(1, 513) = 89.34, p < .001$. The valid number of cases in the analysis was 515, with 86 in Cluster 1 (pathological lying) and 429 in Cluster 2 (nonpathological lying). Thus, the cluster analysis indicated that pathological lying, based on the Four Fs, may represent approximately 5.99% of the sample. With this analysis, the prevalence of pathological lying ranges from approximately 6% to 13%. The 6% to 8% estimate may be a more accurate and conservative estimate of the prevalence of pathological lying in the population-based on cluster analysis and the sensitivity and specificity criteria of the DQ-5. However, this lower estimate should not discount the possibility of self-report reflecting the presence of an actual condition. Some people who experience symptoms of psychopathology are aware of their symptoms and condition.

Compulsivity, Motivation, and the Hydra Hypothesis

We found that pathological liars reported compulsive features to their lying. People in the pathological lying group indicated that their lying was out of their control and that they felt less anxious after telling a lie more than those in the nonpathological lying group. Regarding motivation, pathological liars also indicated that they told lies for no reason more than people in the nonpathological lying group. Lastly, we found support for the Hydra hypothesis, in that pathological liars indicated a greater propensity for their lies to grow from an initial one compared with nonpathological liars. Case studies and another assessment study that we conducted, which are discussed in Chapter 7, align with this finding.

Pathological Liars Versus Prolific Liars

On the basis of the previously discussed theory of pathological lying, pathological liars would be a distinct group of people who not only tell an excessive amount of lies but also show features of impaired functioning, feeling pain, and lies being fatal. Within the nonpathological lying sample, a group of prolific liars was identified, people who told three or more lies per day. When comparing this group with the pathological lying group, we found that pathological liars reported greater impaired functioning, feeling pain, and danger from telling lies compared with the prolific liars. Further, we found that pathological liars indicated a greater propensity to tell lies within their everyday life, as indicated by scores on the Lying in Everyday Situations scale, compared with the prolific liars.

Others' Perceptions of Pathological Liars

In addition to surveying nonpathological liars about their lying behavior, we asked them if they had known anyone whom they considered to be a pathological liar, and if so, would they be willing to report on that person. Overall, and somewhat surprisingly, people's accounts of pathological liars matched fairly similarly to the actual accounts of pathological liars. Participants estimated that people they knew to be pathological liars told an average of 10 lies per day and mode of five lies per day. Most participants indicated that the onset was in adolescence and the person had been lying for longer than 6 months. Participants indicated that the person's lies resulted in impaired functioning, mostly in social relationships. Lastly, participants indicated that the person's lies were significantly distressing and dangerous.

EXPERIENCES WITH PATHOLOGICAL LIARS

Relatedly, we recently conducted another study with some other colleagues that was aimed at further exploring people's interactions with pathological liars and aspects of those interactions (Hart, Beech, & Curtis, 2022). We hypothesized that most people have interacted with someone whom they believed was a pathological liar at some point in their life. We recruited 251 participants and asked them whether they had ever interacted with a pathological, compulsive, or habitual liar. The participants were then asked four open-ended questions about various aspects of the lies. Statements were classified by two independent raters who displayed a high interrater reliability (between 87% and 100%). Our findings were that a majority of people (91%) reported they had interacted with a pathological liar. Similar to the findings from Curtis and Hart (2020), participants estimated that pathological liars told about 10 lies per day, whereas most other people tell two lies per day. Participants also believed that a distinction of pathological liars is the number of lies they tell per day—that it is telling nine or more lies per day.

Furthermore, participants believed that pathological liars tell lies for no specific reason or motive (Hart, Beech, & Curtis, 2022). All participants indicated that pathological liars told lies for self-serving reasons rather than the benefit of others. Other findings indicated that participants believed pathological liars to lie about themselves, that their lying had negative outcomes on social and emotional functioning, and that the lying affected half of the participants emotionally and socially. When asked how the participants knew that a pathological liar was lying, more than half indicated that they knew because the lies were improbable. A smaller group (23%) indicated that they learned about the lies through evidence.

PSYCHOLINGUISTIC ANALYSIS OF PATHOLOGICAL LYING

Because pathological lying has yet to be recognized as a formal psychiatric diagnosis, some pathological liars have discussed their behavior on blogs and forums. We, with another colleague, examined blog and forum writings to better understand aspects of pathological lying (Curtis et al., 2021). We analyzed the narratives of 22 pathological liars, 21 people from a normative group, and normative data published by Pennebaker and colleagues (2015) using Linguistic Inquiry and Word Count (LIWC; Pennebaker et al., 2015). We compared four LIWC analysis variables: analytic, clout, authentic, and tone.

Our findings revealed significance for all four variables. The writings of pathological liars were less analytic, had less clout, and had less tone but were more authentic compared with a normative sample. Lower scores on analytic, clout, and tone can be suggestive of a more informal or personal style and revealing of greater distress (Pennebaker et al., 2015). Higher authentic scores are typically suggestive of a more honest, open, or self-disclosing style (Pennebaker et al., 2015). We also compared pathological liars' writings with the writings of normative liars across the four LIWC variables, finding pathological liars to be less analytic. Our findings not only highlight the existence of pathological lying through blogs and forums but also reveal that pathological liars appear to be forthcoming about their distress from lying. A number of pathological liars would post questions about how to get help, how to stop lying, ways to fix their relationships, or just to get support. It is likely that the failure to formally recognize pathological lying and the absence of specific treatments have led people to seek help through online platforms.

RECOGNITION OF PATHOLOGICAL LYING

Pathological lying has long been recognized by many prominent psychiatrists and psychologists from various countries. However, different languages, various names, and differing definitions have likely led to it being overlooked or not included within major nosological systems. Even so, there has been a plethora of evidence in case studies alone to suggest the recognition of pathological lying as a distinct diagnostic entity. In addition to these clinical examples, there exists empirical investigations as early as 1915 (by Healy & Healy), although these studies are few. A reemergence of interest in pathological lying has led to research on neuroimaging of brain matter and brain structures found within a pathological lying sample. Although this is an important area of research for understanding pathological lying, there remains more to be examined. As Spence (2005) rightfully noted, the current neuroscience research on pathological lying has yet to determine whether brain structure precedes lying behavior.

Our large-scale, theory-driven study provided more evidence of the distinctiveness of pathological lying and has laid the foundation for the classification of pathological lying. We suggested features and markers of pathological lying that can be clinically assessed and studied within the laboratory. Given past definitions, clinical cases, and research findings, we suggest an updated definition of pathological lying, one that aligns with major nosological systems, defining it as follows:

> A persistent, pervasive, and often compulsive pattern of excessive lying behavior leading to clinically significant impairment of functioning in social, occupational, or other areas, causing marked distress, and posing a risk to the self or others, occurring for longer than a six-month period. (Curtis & Hart, 2020b, p. 63)

Recent research and an updated definition brings promise to better understanding pathological lying and for research efforts. We agree with Spence's (2005) criticism of Yang et al.'s (2005) classification of pathological lying and hope that our definition and classification remedies this concern by offering a unified definition and parameters for classification. In the following chapters, we examine other means of assessment and suggest diagnostic criteria for pathological lying.

6

Pathological Lying on the Couch

Psychotherapy is a place for confession and secrets. Patients confide in professional strangers and share their deepest pains, thoughts, and behaviors that have not been vocalized to any other person in the world. Psychotherapy is structured in a manner to facilitate full disclosure through means such as confidentiality and an active listener who is fully equipped to handle any story, information, or emotions that are presented. Psychotherapy is built on a foundation of trust and open communication. So, how might a therapist assess, diagnose, and even treat a person whose sole problem involves being a pathological liar? Does this apparent paradox of a patient providing misinformation to determine a patient's problem not fly in the face of the core structure of psychotherapy? Furthermore, do people even lie in therapy, and if so, why? Why would anyone spend time and resources for psychotherapy only to deceive the therapist?

https://doi.org/10.1037/0000305-006
Pathological Lying: Theory, Research, and Practice, by D. A. Curtis and C. L. Hart

The question about lying in psychotherapy is somewhat novel and rarely on the radar of most psychologists and mental health professionals. In fact, the impetus for one of us to begin studying deception, specifically within psychotherapeutic contexts, was based on an experience in clinical training. During practicum, one of us had seen a patient who had entered counseling for relational and trust concerns. Essentially, the patient had cheated on his significant other, and she found out by secretly accessing his phone. She was angry and hurt by being cheated on and lied to. So, the patient agreed to therapy to work on ways to be more honest within his relationship. A couple of sessions in, the patient was asked a question about lying behavior, and he responded that he never lies. The therapist was confused and taken aback, especially given that the presenting problem centered on deceptive practices with a significant other. This case was subsequently presented within a practicum classroom setting. Lo and behold, all other students in the class reported having no experiences with patient deception. The sum total of clinical training received in patient deception was some worthwhile questions and brief advice that spanned less than 5 minutes. Patient deception was not an area that was part of formal clinical training and appeared not to be an area that doctoral students often thought about (at least students in this situation). The lack of clinical training in patient deception was not a function of a poor-quality training program but represented the field as a whole. It was later discovered that this experience was not unique, in that therapists have experiences with patient deception yet receive little to no training in the area.

In 2011, Kottler and Carlson published a unique book that captured the accounts of various therapists' experiences and recollections with patient deception (discovered deception). Within the book, various therapists, seasoned masters to neophytes, shared a range of experiences in working with patient deception. Some patients made false allegations of a therapist soliciting sex (Carlson, 2011) and others fabricated an entire therapy persona (Grzegorek, 2011). What is evident from the collection of therapists' experiences is that deception in therapy occurs and most therapists have not received much training within this area. In fact, one of the therapists that reflected on a case had stated "we are rarely trained to recognize when we are being deceived" (Helm, 2011, p. 82).

In 2015, we published a study about psychotherapists' beliefs, attitudes, and experiences with client deception (Curtis & Hart, 2015). From across 421 American Psychological Association internship sites, we recruited 112 participants. Participants ranged in age from 25 to 69 years, represented various ethnicities, endorsed a variety of theoretical frameworks, and had a wide range of psychotherapy experience (from under 1 year up to 40 years). We found that the majority of psychotherapists reported minimal training in three areas: general exposure to deception, training with client deception, and with deception detection. Interestingly, psychotherapists in forensics report, on average, only slightly more training in deception (Dickens & Curtis, 2019). Forensic psychotherapists indicated reading a moderate amount of deception literature, receiving moderate training, and little to moderate training with deception detection (Dickens & Curtis, 2019). The same finding emerges when we give workshop presentations to psychotherapists (many seasoned practitioners). Clinicians have often reported to one of us that the most training they have received in patient deception came from the workshop provided. Thus, if training is minimal to nonexistent, then it is likely that practitioners are not prepared to work with pathological liars.

Given the lack of training within deception in psychotherapy, we present research and literature pertaining to deception within psychotherapy. We first examine the core assumption of honesty within psychotherapy and the beliefs that practitioners hold about deception. We then discuss an overview of research findings regarding the frequency of patient deception, types of lies, and topics of deception. The research findings provide a basis for understanding normative lying within psychotherapy and distinguish between pathological lying. We then discuss our recent research findings on psychotherapists' clinical experiences with patients who were pathological liars.

HONESTY ASSUMPTION

Psychotherapy operates on a major assumption: that people will be honest. In fact, the entire process, from assessment to treatment, would be compromised if a patient were to be completely dishonest. Consider the case of a patient who fabricated a psychotherapy persona with the intent of seeing if he could fool the therapist (Grzegorek, 2011). The case was a 20-year-old who sought counseling at university counseling services. After several psychotherapy sessions, the patient entered the final session and laughed. When queried, he stated that he lied about everything. The patient told the therapist that he liked to have fun with people and wanted to see if he could fool someone who committed years to studying human behavior. In this case, all parts of the therapeutic process were based on the information provided, which was all false information. Thus, the only goal achieved was that of the patient, who likely was chasing duping delight, trying to see if he could successfully dupe a master of human behavior. He did. Was he a pathological liar? It is possible—he certainly lied excessively. However, it would be important to assess whether the patient's lying behavior was only contextualized to the psychotherapeutic context or permeated other aspects of his life, causing him impairment in functioning, distress, and other risks.

Although somewhat unconventional in a scientific book, let us consider a poem about deception in psychotherapy. Yu (2009) wrote a poem about a pathological liar's experience with psychotherapy and an apology to her therapist:

> Attic office, turquoise carpet, rock fountain on the end table, its drowned gurgle—I admit at first these filled me with contempt, and the Madame Alexanders in the pram made me uneasy. But I stayed out of pity for your heart-embroidered vest and your eagerness as you leaned toward me, pen poised above a clipboard.
>
> When you asked about my marriage, I lied. My job, that too. When you asked for a dream, I confess I gave my mother's, the one that woke her coughing, thinking she'd choked on her sister's tangled, hip-length hair. Truth is, I'm an only child
>
> But after you pulled the *Encyclopedia of Dreams* From the shelf below the Hummels and decoded the throat of hair as an estrangement, spitting a little in your pleasure, I invented others, presents I brought each Thursday at II. They fell from my lips as glossy and

inevitable as coupons from the Sunday paper, and you translated them like fortunes in a dead language.

> *A gold bracelet in a well: an old friend will call. A cut on my ring finger: desire for a lover. A child crying on the doorstep of an empty house: some unfinished task. Happiness: unspoken sorrow.*

I wish I'd given you the real one, the only one I do dream each long, blank night: my teeth crumbling, crown and cementum cracking.

I should I have told you what I really wanted when I woke at dawn, gasping—a gold tooth to replace a molar, just one, anchored in my jaw, slender threads of gold running deep to touch bone, a gold tooth hidden in the back of my mouth near the beginning of words, like a secret or a blunt pain I could prod with my tongue, a pain I could test and be sure of. (Yu, 2009, pp. 461–462)[1]

This poem highlights the importance of the truth assumption in therapy. The ending denotes the regret of not being honest within therapy and an apology to the therapist for not being forthcoming with the actual concerns. The poem illustrates that the various lies told to the therapist provided a disservice by hiding the patient's actual concerns.

Honesty within psychotherapy is so strongly presumed that it may not even be discussed. In some cases, therapists may discuss the expectation of honesty at the onset of therapy. The strong assumption of honesty within psychotherapy often produces a truth bias for most therapists (Curtis, 2013; Kottler & Carlson, 2011). As we discuss more fully, this bias serves a useful function because most people are honest most of the time within psychotherapy (Curtis & Hart, 2020a). In fact, most social interactions tend to be honest (Bond & DePaulo, 2006; Levine, 2014b, 2020; Serota et al., 2010; Serota & Levine, 2015). However, deception in psychotherapeutic contexts does occur, and when it does, most therapists report a range of emotional reactions and having a lack of training (Kottler & Carlson, 2011).

---

[1]From "The Compulsive Liar Apologizes to Her Therapist for Certain Fabrications and Omissions," by J. Yu, 2009 (Fall–Winter), *TriQuarterly, 135–136*, pp. 461–462. Copyright 2009 by Northwestern University. Reprinted with permission.

There is an exception to this rule. The words expressed by a psychopathology teacher on the first day of class are still embedded in the memory of one of the authors. He said of patients, echoing the television character Gregory House, "Everyone lies, I just need to know what they are lying about." His primary vocation was working at correctional facilities. This psychologist was demonstrating the other side of the coin, the lie bias, in assuming that most patients lie most of the time. Beyond anecdote, the lie bias has been found to reside more strongly with forensic practitioners (Dickens & Curtis, 2019).

PINOCCHIO ON THE COUCH

Although Pinocchio never sought psychotherapy for his woes, lying can be found within therapeutic contexts. Unfortunately, there is no such thing as a Pinocchio's nose, or a singular consistent behavior that reliably indicates dishonesty (Vrij, 2008). Kottler and Carlson (2011) provided a great starting point for understanding therapists' accounts of deception within psychotherapy. Along with a lack of training, clinicians reported feeling angry, confused, and surprised. Expanding on therapists' personal stories of being duped, we were broadly interested in clinicians' experiences, beliefs, and attitudes toward patient deception. What do practitioners think deceptive behavior looks like when it presents in therapy and what attitudes are harbored toward those who lie to a therapist? Thus, the previously referenced study we published in 2015 was developed to explore these areas. Specifically, we were interested in assessing whether practitioners possessed a specific advantage when it came to knowledge about deceptive cues. In addition to this, we were interested in learning about therapists' attitudes toward patients who lie in therapy.

Overall, there were two major findings from our study: Psychotherapists have a number of inaccurate beliefs about cues to deception, and they possess several negative attitudes toward patients who lie (Curtis & Hart, 2015). Practitioners held the belief that patients decrease eye contact when they lie. The belief that people avert their gaze when they lie is a common erroneous belief that tends to be strongly endorsed cross-culturally (Global Deception Research Team, 2006). Practitioners endorsed a number of other stereotypical and nondiagnostic beliefs about deception cues. In addition to looking away, therapists believed that when patients lie they tend to move more frequently (hands, feet, shrugs, postural shifts, eye blinks). These beliefs are often associated with the stereotypical belief that liars are nervous or anxious and fidget or move more. Vrij (2008) provided three explanations for beliefs about the liar stereotype. One reason is that lying is associated with moral turpitude and should cause people to feel nervous and ashamed when lying, looking away and fidgeting. Another explanation was that liars are often portrayed in popular media and film to avert their gaze and show anxious behaviors. The third explanation Vrij (2008) put forth was that when people are accused of being liars they may respond with nervousness, even if they are honest. Although practitioners pay attention to nonverbal behaviors, most of these deception cues tend to be unreliable or nondiagnostic when detecting deception (Vrij et al., 2019). Psychotherapists are not alone in their beliefs. Law enforcement professionals tend to hold similar inaccurate beliefs about deception cues (Bogaard et al., 2016).

Our other important discovery was that psychotherapists held a number of negative attitudes toward patients who lie (Curtis & Hart, 2015). Practitioners indicated that discovering a patient was being deceptive would lead to liking the patient less, having less of a desire to interact with the patient, being less enthusiastic about working with the patient, being less trusting of the patient, thinking less positively about the patient, seeing the patient as insincere, and thinking more negatively about the patient. Further, patients who lied in psychotherapy were judged to be less successful, less compliant, less pleasant, less likeable, and less adjusted.

Taken together, the concern is that a lack of training in deception and holding inaccurate beliefs about deceptive behavior may lead to a therapist assuming a patient is lying when they are not. For example, a patient who is looking away could be wrongfully judged as lying even though they were showing respect to the therapist or feeling ashamed about some personal experience. The major concern is not just an inaccurate assessment of the veracity of a patient's behavior but that consequently the therapist will hold negative attitudes toward the patient who is viewed as a liar. So, what can be done and how might these findings affect work with pathological liars? We discuss implications and recommendations for clinical practice in Chapter 9, but essentially therapists should pursue more training, seek the function of the lie(s), and be aware of one's bias and attitudes toward lies and liars.

LYING ON THE COUCH

It is clear that some therapists have been duped by patients. It also stands to reason that there are therapists who have been lied to by a patient and never discovered the deception. Does this mean that lying is a frequent occurrence within psychotherapy? Does lying on the proverbial couch mean telling your therapist lies? We discuss two studies that examined the frequency of patient deception.

Blanchard and Farber (2016) recruited 547 adult psychotherapy patients to participate in an online survey. Participants were provided with a list of 58 topics and asked to select the topics they recalled being dishonest about within psychotherapy. If participants had selected more than one topic, they were also asked to rate the extent that they were dishonest about each of the ones they selected. In addition to this, the researchers had a second section that was designed to obtain qualitative information. The researchers found a majority of participants (93%) had been deceptive with their therapists. The sample recalled lying about 4,616 topics, and on average each patient lied in eight categories. Further, they found that around 73% of participants reported at least one lie about therapy-related topics (e.g., "pretending to like my therapist's comments or suggestions"). Participants endorsed a range of topics that they recalled lying about in psychotherapy. The topic endorsed by most participants (54%) was minimizing how bad they felt, followed by minimizing severity of symptoms (39%) and thoughts of suicide (31%). Farber and colleagues (2019) reported that in a second study, they found some of the most commonly reported topics of ongoing dishonesty consisted of client sexual desires or fantasies (34%), details of sex life (33%), and suicidal thoughts (21%).

We also conducted a study on the frequency of deception in psychotherapy (Curtis & Hart, 2020a). Our methods were different from Blanchard and Farber's (2016) approach, as we used deceptive vignettes and explicitly asked people to report on their deceptive behavior within psychotherapy. We recruited 252 college students, and 91 of them indicated having been or currently being in psychotherapy. Participants were provided with two sets of deception vignettes (therapy and general) that contained six types of deceptions (e.g., omission, falsification, white lie) for a total of 12 vignettes. For each vignette, participants responded to several questions (e.g., "have you ever made this type of statement to a therapist?"). Following the vignettes, we explicitly asked participants to report on their use of deception in psychotherapy. Across all vignettes, we found that 89% of participants indicated using at least one type of deception. When explicitly asked about the total number of times a participant had been deceptive in therapy, we found that about 86% indicated they had been deceptive at least once. Participants reported telling about two lies ($M = 1.59$) within a 50-minute session, with zero as the most frequent response. Thus, we found a positively skewed distribution of lies told within psychotherapy. Most people reported telling no lies within a 50-minute therapy session, and a smaller group of people indicated telling many more lies. Although most people who have been to psychotherapy have lied, it is not a frequent event. We also found that if participants lied, it was more likely to be during the initial meeting with a therapist compared with subsequent meetings.

Along with discovering that most people do not often lie in therapy, we also explored the types of lies used. We found white lies, with the intent to protect the therapist, were endorsed more than any of the other types of lies. For example, a patient may claim that psychotherapy is going really well when it has not been or that it is leading to a number of positive life changes when, in fact, nothing in the person's life is different. Patients may also tell the therapist that they like them when they are indifferent or do not like the therapist. These white lies are told for the sake of protecting or benefitting the therapist.

Our findings paint an interesting picture of deception in psychotherapy. Lying in psychotherapy is not a ubiquitous phenomenon in which patients are maliciously trying to undermine therapists. It is quite the opposite. Most people are not lying often in psychotherapy. When people do lie, it is likely to be early on, in the initial meeting of the therapist.

Further, the lies that are told tend to be told with the intent of protecting the therapist (white lies). Taken together, therapists may hold negative attitudes toward patients who lie in psychotherapy, but ironically, the few instances of deception are told with the intent of protecting the therapist. However, not all deception in therapy consists of white lies or occurs with a relatively low frequency. Keep in mind the curve, in that there is a smaller group of people who are lying quite often. Let's consider those cases.

PATHOLOGICAL LYING ON THE COUCH

I'm a textbook pathological liar. I never really saw my lying as a problem. But I've come to realize, that I think this pathological lying is making my life more stressful and miserable than it could be. I've told so many lies to different people, it's impossible for me to keep track of them all, and now have the notoriety of being a liar. Obviously I'd like to wipe this reputation clean, so I why I'm here. A lot of the lies I tell serve no real purpose. I'll lie about things like. What I had for breakfast. Things which REALLY don't matter in the slightest, but I lie about them anyway. It's uncontrollable, I don't really think before saying them. . . . It's compulsive. I have a habit of manipulating family members into pitying me, which leads to them doing things for me, such as letting me live with them. I lied about having Asperger's syndrome, and then attempted suicide, although I didn't care if I died or not. It was purely a lie to make my mum think I was depressed so she would feel bad and let me stay with her for a while. I know I'm a "bad" person. But I would like help with this, any tips? I'd love to go get therapy, But I'd LIE. lol And I got falsely diagnosed with AsPD not long ago, so I refuse to go back.

—Person who identified as a pathological liar

I have been lying since I was a kid. Back in school I would lie about things I did or people I [k]new just to be liked by the popular kids. Now I am married with children and the lying continues. I lie about stupid things, for example things I did that day. The bigger lies have

gotten us into financial problems and me into legal problems where
I almost went to prison. I have been in therapy for some yrs now for
this problem among others.

—Person who identified as a compulsive liar

Anecdotally, we have provided various case studies, clinical examples,
and experiences of pathological lying reported within blogs. In looking at
the lie frequency data, one robust finding tends to surface: the ski slope of
the positively skewed distribution of lying. The lying distribution has been
found in high school students (Levine et al., 2013), a large sample of the
U.S. population (Serota et al., 2010), a large sample in the United Kingdom
(Serota & Levine, 2015), and in a Japanese sample (Daiku et al., 2021).
This distribution was what facilitated the exploration into pathological
lying. Along with strong evidence for the positively skewed distribution
in various samples, it has also been recorded within the few studies that
have examined lying in psychotherapy.

Recall that our study on deception in psychotherapy (Curtis & Hart,
2020a) found the positively skewed distribution with regard to the number
of lies told within a 50-minute therapy session (see Figure 6.1). We suggested that the smaller percentage of people who tell numerous lies in
psychotherapy needs further investigation, in that these individuals
could represent pathological lying or some other psychopathology. Using
the Serota and colleagues (2010) cutoff of five or more lies, about 8% of
patients belong to this category. Using the three or more lies cutoff criteria, as done in our pathological lying study (Curtis & Hart, 2020b), we
find about 11% of the sample fit this category. The group of people who
told numerous lies in psychotherapy did not reveal any significant differences across demographic variables (e.g., age, sex, education).

In their book, *Secrets and Lies in Psychotherapy*, Farber and colleagues
(2019) reexamined topics lied about from the Blanchard and Farber (2016)
study. Specifically, they reported that their distribution of topics lied about
was positively skewed, similar to the prolific liar findings from Serota and
colleagues (2010) and Serota and Levine (2015). They found about 6%
of participants who indicated lying about 20 or more topics (of 58 total
topics; see Figure 6.2).

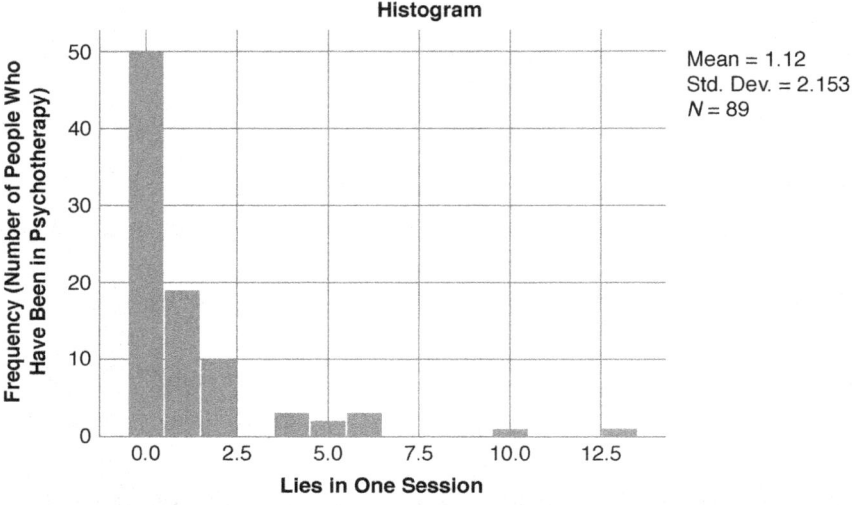

Figure 6.1

Findings of the distribution of lies told within one therapy session. Data from Curtis and Hart (2020a).

Farber and colleagues (2019) referred to the 6% as "prolific therapy liars" (p. 132). They indicated that this group not only reported lying about more topics but also telling bigger lies. Compared with the other participants, they found no racial or gender differences. However, they found that the group of prolific therapy liars were about 5 years younger and were twice as likely to report that traumatic experiences was the reason they entered therapy.

These two studies were aimed at getting a general sense of lying frequency within psychotherapy. However, both studies reveal the same trend found in other lie frequency studies—a positive skew. A smaller group of people tell many lies. It can only be inferred that some of these individuals consist of pathological liars. On the basis of historical clinical accounts, it is evident that clinicians have worked with pathological liars. To get a more complete picture of pathological lying within clinical contexts, we discuss a study we conducted with practitioners.

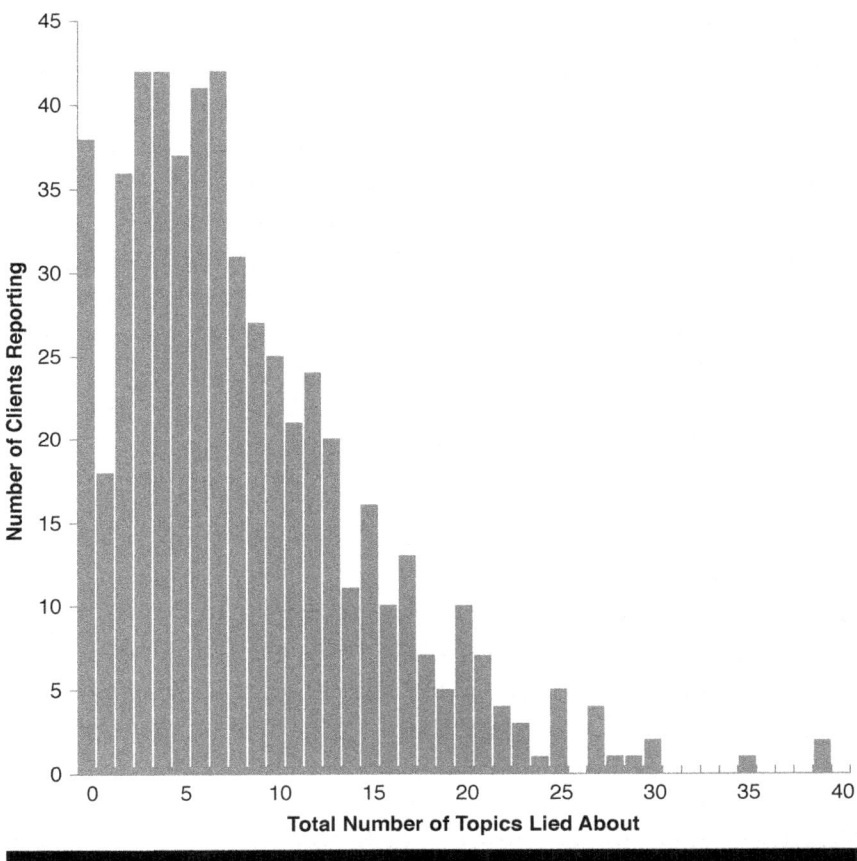

Figure 6.2

Distribution analysis of Blanchard and Farber (2016) data. Adapted from *Secrets and Lies in Psychotherapy* (p. 133), by B. Farber, M. Blanchard, and M. Love, 2019, American Psychological Association (https://doi.org/10.1037/0000128-000). Copyright 2019 by the American Psychological Association.

PATHOLOGICAL LYING: PSYCHOTHERAPISTS' EXPERIENCES AND ABILITY TO DIAGNOSE

As there have been widely documented cases of pathological lying within clinical settings, we sought to investigate practitioners' experiences with pathological lying (Curtis & Hart, 2021c). Specifically, we wanted to assess practitioners' beliefs about pathological lying being a distinct diagnostic entity, examine their experiences in working with pathological lying, and determine their ability to accurately diagnose pathological lying. We discuss the ability to accurately diagnose pathological lying more in Chapter 8.

We sent emails to practitioners via the Association of Psychology Postdoctoral and Internship Centers, the Texas State Board of Examiners of Psychologists email list, and the Texas Society of Psychiatric Physicians. A total of 295 participants completed our study. The majority of participants were doctoral-level practitioners and licensed psychologists. There were other mental health practitioners who participated, including licensed psychological associates licensed professional counselors, licensed marriage and family therapists, and psychiatrists. Participants held a wide range of experience, having provided counseling or psychotherapy for less than a year to 54 years.

The first major question we asked practitioners was whether they believed that pathological lying should be considered a diagnostic entity. More than half of the clinicians (52%) indicated that pathological lying should be considered a diagnostic entity. Most practitioners (74%) indicated having worked with a patient who was considered to be a pathological liar. In more accounts, practitioners indicated that their patients were considered pathological liars because the patient explicitly discussed difficulties with excessive lying behavior and other information provided. Although a smaller percentage, some clinicians (20%) reported that some of their patients' presenting problem was pathological lying. When asked to estimate caseload, the majority of clinicians reported that pathological lying consisted of less than 10% of their cases.

The majority of the practitioners (86%) reported that their patients, those identified as pathological liars, had lied to them during their work together. They estimated that their patients told an average of 11 lies per day, with the most frequent response being five lies told per day. Similar to the other findings of lie frequency, a positive skew emerged (see Figure 6.3). Among pathological liars in psychotherapy, some were reported to tell many more lies than others. Interestingly, these estimates of practitioners

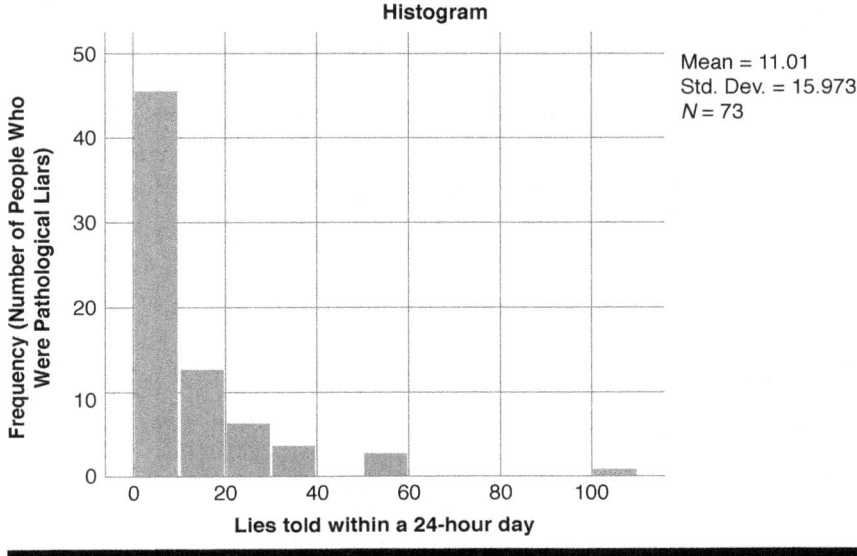

Histogram

Mean = 11.01
Std. Dev. = 15.973
N = 73

Figure 6.3

Findings of the distribution of lies told from pathological liars in psychotherapy. Data from Curtis and Hart (2021c).

closely resemble that of the general population with regard to people they identified as being pathological liars (Curtis & Hart, 2020b).

In addition to reported frequency, practitioners indicated that their patients' lies impaired functioning and caused significant distress. Similar to our previously reported findings from the reports of pathological lairs, we found that therapists stated that their patients had been telling excessive lies for more than 6 months and that the onset was generally in adolescence. Clinicians also largely indicated that their patients' lies tended to grow from an initial lie. One area where practitioners did not show a clear level of agreement pertained to whether the patient's lying behavior was outside of their control and that their lies were told for no reason. The lack of a clear position may be related to some therapists believing that behavioral change is possible and within a patient's control and that patients' lies serve some function and are therefore being told for a reason. However, we did not fully explore this within our research.

LYING AND PATHOLOGICAL LYING
WITHIN PSYCHOTHERAPY

Many people have lied to a therapist. However, most people are generally honest within psychotherapy. When people do lie in therapy, it is usually telling white lies to protect the therapist. In some instances, patients may lie to minimize symptoms or about their suicidal ideation. Within the population of people who seek psychotherapy, there is a smaller group of people who tell numerous lies. Some of these patients represent pathological liars. Pathological lying is not a frequent occurrence within psychotherapy. Many people who identified as pathological liars in our study (Curtis & Hart, 2021c) did not have a formal diagnosis. This likely indicates that they had not sought mental health services. Along with these individuals, there are people who post blogs and videos seeking support and help for their pathological lying (Curtis & Hart, 2021b). People who engage in pathological lying may seek psychotherapy services because of the impact of their lying on their relationships. In some cases, therapy may be viewed as the last straw, or it has been family mandated. However, the lack of formal recognition of pathological lying as a diagnostic entity may prevent some people from seeking therapeutic services. In the case of the person quoted previously (who identified as a pathological liar), the person was inaccurately diagnosed with antisocial personality disorder, which deterred the person from returning to psychotherapy.

7

Assessment

The process of psychotherapy is not cryptic or mystical. It is fairly simple. The process is essentially the same as the practice of medicine. If you have ever broken a bone or been injured, then you know this process well. A person may go to the emergency department where there is paperwork, an interview of sorts, and then maybe get an X-ray of the injured area. Then the physician communicates the problem, as identified by the various pieces of information. Last, the broken bone is treated with a cast, and the individual may receive pain medication.

The same process can even be seen when taking your vehicle to an auto mechanic. Your mechanic conducts an assessment, which includes an interview, asking about the problem. Then the mechanic tells you the diagnosis or problem(s) with your vehicle. Lastly, the treatment consists of fixing or replacing the parts.

https://doi.org/10.1037/0000305-007
Pathological Lying: Theory, Research, and Practice, by D. A. Curtis and C. L. Hart

In psychotherapy, the same process unfolds. A psychotherapist's role typically includes providing assessments, diagnosis, and treatment through psychotherapy (American Psychological Association [APA], 2006, 2020a, 2020b). The process is simply

Assessment → Diagnosis → Treatment.

The challenge lies in accurately assessing the problem. If the assessment is faulty, then the rest of the process is compromised. To guard against this concern, the APA (2020b) has organized various task force workgroups over the years to work on and publicize guidelines for psychological assessment and evaluation. The woes of clinical practice and challenges of accurate assessment are exemplified in the sobering work of Paul Meehl and David Rosenhan. There is no greater learning than to have to wrestle with research and information that directly challenges the very fabric of your profession. One of the most uncomfortable yet rewarding moments of graduate education for one of us was being presented with the work of Meehl (1954). Meehl's work largely discussed the concerns of clinical and statistical methods of prediction, in that statistical methods outperform clinical methods. He made the case that clinical judgments are unreliable and prone to the errors of human bias. He asserted that simple statistical calculations would allow clinicians to make more accurate diagnoses than their clinical judgment ever would. It may be easy for a practitioner to become defensive in response to Meehl's findings, as they seek to justify their use of clinical judgment. It has prompted others to rely on psychometrically sound assessments to aid in clinical decisions.

About 19 years after Meehl's (1954) seminal work, David Rosenhan (1973) published his findings that largely highlighted concerns of clinical judgments. In his first study, Rosenhan sent eight mentally healthy people to seek admission into 12 psychiatric hospitals. All pseudo-patients feigned broad symptoms of hearing unclear voices during their admission process. They were all admitted and provided a diagnosis of schizophrenia, except one, manic-depressive psychosis. Immediately after admission, all ceased reporting symptoms. Despite their normal behavior and lack of symptoms, all patients were forced to take antipsychotic medications and were kept in the hospital for an average of 19 days. Thus, he found that practitioners were largely biased to inaccurately diagnose pseudo-patients with a psychological disorder when they did not have one, or a false positive. In the second part of the study, Rosenhan found evidence in the opposite direction, in that practitioners and psychiatric nurses believed actual patients to be pseudo-patients when no pseudo-patients were sent. That is, they potentially failed to detect psychopathology when psychopathology may have existed. In sum, Rosenhan's findings revealed that practitioners may be prone to confirmation bias. Increasing accuracy in assessment is often important for medical professionals, mental health practitioners, and even forensic practitioners who are interested in detecting deception. Further, if a patient is deceptive, then this directly challenges the entire process. "If a patient were to fabricate life events or intentionally withhold critical information, then assessment, diagnosis, and treatment could be compromised" (Curtis, 2021a, p. 803).

DETECTING DECEPTION

When it comes to detecting deception, similar issues of assessment and human decision making are found. There are two overarching means by which deception detection is categorized: human and mechanical/assisted. Human detection of deception largely consists of strategies or approaches that people use without reliance or assistance on technology or other instruments. Mechanical or assisted methods consist of those technologies, instruments, devices, or tests that provide additional information that helps people in veracity judgments. There are several books that unpack the various approaches to detect deception and research on the effectiveness of each approach (e.g., Granhag & Strömwall, 2004; Granhag et al., 2015; Levine, 2020; Vrij, 2008), and therefore we provide only an overview of human and mechanical/assisted methods to highlight some of the ways that people assess deceptive behavior. Specific attention is given to psychologists' and other mental health practitioners' ability to detect deception.

Human Ability

The research findings from human deception detectors largely resembles what Meehl (1954) found, in that human judgments are typically not much better than chance in detecting deception. One of the most cited meta-analytic findings of the accuracy of human judges to detect deception is the work of Bond and DePaulo (2006). They collected and analyzed 206 deception detection studies, containing 4,435 senders of deception and 24,483 judges of deception (Bond & DePaulo, 2006). The judges were people who were briefly exposed to unfamiliar people and asked to make veracity judgments without assistance from mechanical aids (e.g., polygraph) or clinical assessments (e.g., MMPI-2). The findings from Bond and DePaulo's meta-analysis were that the accuracy of truth–lie judgments was 54%, with 61% accuracy with truth judgments and 47% accuracy with lie judgments.

What about psychologists or mental health professionals? Are professionals any better at detecting deception? Briggs (1992) examined vocational counselors' abilities to detect deception by randomly assigning 40 participants to 20 counselors. The counselors did not know that half of the participants were informed to lie and the other half were instructed to be honest. Every counselor conducted 15-minute interviews with each person—one who lied and one who was honest. Briggs found that counselors had an 85% accuracy rate, in which honest clients were identified with 90% accuracy and deceptive clients with 80% accuracy.

Ekman et al. (1999) examined psychologists' abilities to detect deception. Of the sample, there were 107 practitioners who were interested in deception, 209 clinical psychologists who did not have a special interest in deception, and 125 academic psychologists. All participants saw 1-minute videos of 10 senders in which half told the truth and half lied. Ekman and colleagues found that clinicians who had an interest in deception performed significantly better than clinical psychologists who had no special interest in deception or academic psychologists.

Although these two studies indicate the prospects of mental health professionals being able to more accurately identify deception, the evidence from a meta-analysis indicated that expert or professional judges do not possess specific advantages in detecting deception (Bond & DePaulo, 2006). Bond and DePaulo's (2006) meta-analysis examined 19 studies of experts, who consisted of "law enforcement personnel, judges, psychiatrists, job interviewers, and auditors—anyone whom deception researchers regard as experts" (p. 229). Their findings revealed that the expert average of lie–truth judgments was approximately 55%.

In an attempt to increase accuracy of deception detection, some companies have promoted their software as a means to improve deception detection through microexpression training (Humintell, 2020; Paul Ekman Group, LLC, 2014). The idea is that by training people to notice fleeting and subtle changes in facial expression (microexpressions), they will be better able to discern who is lying and who is telling the truth. To test the claims that microexpression training can increase deception detection, Curtis (2021a) conducted a study to examine whether the software improved deception detection compared with a control group of people who watched a cognitive behavior therapy video. Although the software improved emotion recognition scores, it did not appear to provide any specific advantages for detecting deception.

Some strategies have been more promising for human deception detection. Hartwig and colleagues (2005, 2006) found that strategic use of evidence improved deception detection accuracy. Specifically, disclosure of evidence later within an interview lead to higher lie-detection accuracy (approximately 68%; Hartwig et al., 2005). Implementing the strategic use of evidence with police trainees were more accurate in detecting deception (approximately 85%; Hartwig et al., 2006). Vrij and colleagues (2006, 2008) developed a deception detection interviewing method designed to impose cognitive load. Ways to impose cognitive load during interviewing may be by asking an interviewee to tell their story in reverse order or by maintaining eye contact during the interview (Vrij et al., 2010). Meta-analytic findings indicated that the cognitive approach yielded increased accuracy of truth and lie detection compared with standard strategies (Vrij et al., 2017). Levine and colleagues (2014) found a method that broke the 90% deception detection barrier and was able to achieve 98% to 100% accuracy. The increased accuracy rates were attributed to specific interviewing methods, using an adapted version of the behavioral analysis interview. However, these findings and methods have been criticized as having theoretical and methodological concerns (Vrij et al., 2015).

Mechanical and Assisted Methods

To aid in lie detection, other methods have been explored. In addition to human behavioral observations, there are three major ways by which people detect deception: (a) physiological responses, (b) speech and writing analysis, and (c) measuring brain activity (Granhag et al., 2015). These methods largely involve technologies, instruments, or tests, which include polygraphs, other physiological measures, brain imaging, speech analysis software, or psychological assessments. Of these methods, the most popular is arguably the polygraph, which is often called the lie detector (Meijer & Verschuere, 2015). The polygraph is not a lie detector; it is a machine that measures physiological processes (e.g., heart rate) and has a long history and association with detecting deception (National Research Council, 2003). Two major interviewing techniques are used with the polygraph: the Control Question Technique (CQT) and the Concealed Information Test (CIT; Lykken, 1957; Meijer & Verschuere, 2015; Reid, 1947). Essentially, the CQT consists of measuring physiological responses to asking control questions compared with responses when asking the relevant questions (or questions of interest). For example, a control question may be about date of birth, and the relevant question may consist of whether a person stabbed a specific victim at a specific time and place. The assumption is that physiological changes would indicate guilt. The CIT is a little different from the CQT, in that it only assesses the details of the incident that would only be known to the police or person who committed a crime. Although the polygraph and these two interviewing methods offer accuracy rates higher than human deception detection, ranging from 59% to 98%, this is still "well below perfection" (Meijer & Verschuere, 2015; National Research Council, 2003, p. 4). The concerns for accuracy are what largely influence decisions of courts holding that the polygraph is inadmissible (Ben-Shakhar et al., 2002; *Daubert v. Merrell Dow Pharmaceuticals, Inc.*, 1993; Vrij, 2008).

Although there have been some investigations on polygraphs and psychopathy (e.g., Lykken, 1978; Patrick & Iacono, 1989; Raskin & Hare, 1978; Verschuere et al., 2006), the literature on pathological lying and polygraphs is scant. Floch (1950) suggested that "the pathological liar certainly will not show any significant reaction to the lie detector test" (p. 652). Psychopathy may not show remorse or may have diminished responses, but our research indicates that pathological liars differ by experiencing pain, guilt, and remorse (Curtis & Hart, 2020b, 2021c). One case study of pseudologia fantastica found that the individual reported guilt and unease (Powell et al., 1983). Thus, pathological liars could very well show physiological changes with the polygraph.

Another method explored has been to examine verbal cues or by conducting linguistic analyses. Verbal analysis has been conducted in three major ways: (a) statement validity analysis (SVA), (b) reality monitoring (RM), and (c) scientific content analysis (SCAN; Vrij, 2015). The premise behind linguistic analysis is that people speak differently when lying than when telling the truth and trying to control speech more when lying is cognitively taxing (Vrij & Mann, 2006). Content analysis entails several steps, usually involving an analysis of the case file, an interview, criteria-based content analysis (CBCA), and a validity checklist (Vrij, 2015). The CBCA and RM have produced accuracy scores around 70% (Vrij, 2015). The SCAN method, although popular, has been criticized for the dearth of empirical support (Bogaard et al., 2021; Vrij, 2015).

Lastly, with the rise in technology, brain imaging has been used to examine lie detection. The brain electrical oscillations signature test was developed as an alternative to the polygraph using measuring brain waves, onset or peaks around 300 to 500 milliseconds or P300 waves (Mukundan et al., 2017). Interviewers may measure brain waves while implementing the CQT or the CIT. Accuracy rates of the P300 with the guilty knowledge test has yielded rates of 88% truth and 82% lie detection (Vrij, 2008). In addition to brain waves, the use of functional magnetic resonance imaging (fMRI) has been explored for deception detection. The accuracy from fMRI studies of deception detection have ranged from 65% to 100% (Ganis, 2015). Although the accuracy rates for brain technologies are much higher than human rates, some authors have raised the question about its applicability within real-world settings and argued the potential dangers of false convictions (Satel & Lilienfeld, 2013). There is no Pinocchio's nose or singular behavior that consistently predicts deception, and there is also no *lie spot*, or a singular area of the brain that consistently reveals deception. There is "no brain region [that] uniquely changes activity when a person lies; each type of lie requires its own set of neural processes" (Satel & Lilienfeld, 2013, p. 91).

REAL-WORLD DETECTION

There are numerous means by which we can detect deception, some offering higher accuracy rates than others, but many of these approaches are not used in everyday situations. The technologically assisted techniques tend to be reserved for academic researchers, some used in forensic settings, or implemented by the military or government agencies. Most people do not subject their significant other and kids to a polygraph when they want to know who ate the last slice of pizza from the refrigerator. Although this is impractical, we also suggest it is not a good practice for maintaining interpersonal relationships. This is certainly the dilemma faced by most therapists because their primary function is not to serve as an interrogator, rooting out every lie from a patient.

So how do most people detect deception in typical world contexts? Park and colleagues (2002) explored this question by recruiting 202 undergraduate students and asking them to recall a recent situation in which they discovered that someone had lied to them. The participants reported using various methods of gathering evidence and confessions. Most deception detection did not occur in the moment or by using verbal and nonverbal cues. Instead, they discovered the deception by gathering information, collateral data, or a confession sometime after the incident (Park et al., 2002).

For most people, this is likely the same method used to discover pathological liars. After being lied to, one may get contradictory evidence or third-party accounts, or the person may even confess. In some of our research on pathological liars, we found that in several instances people would either get caught or confess their lies in attempts to seek help (Curtis & Hart, 2021a, 2021b). From our blog study of pathological lying, one anonymous person who was in a relationship with a pathological liar indicated that the

> web of lies unraveled and I slowly started discovering that a lot of the things [the person] told me weren't true. I started to connect the dots and finally realized what happened to me: I had a relationship with a compulsive liar.

Additionally, there are instances in which pathological liars realize the harm that their lies may be causing and confess their lies. For example, an anonymous individual who lied to their physician stated,

> I realised I'm a compulsive liar. And I went and told my doctor, with the hope that my courage would be rewarded; that my lie would be wiped clean off the record and I could go back to the [medication] I was on, but, no. I can never go down that road again.

Another anonymous person worried their marriage was "heading for divorce because of my compulsive lying! . . . I have finally found a therapist that I can probably trust. Any suggestions of what I can do? I'm hoping to be placed on my meds again soon also. Help!!!"

CLINICAL ASSESSMENTS

Clinically, most people who seek out psychotherapeutic services are feeling pain, with the exception of those who are mandated. From the evidence gathered, most people who engage in pathological lying experience pain and remorse; many are desperate and asking for help. People who realize that their lying is having a negative effect on the ones they love may seek psychotherapy as a means to save or restore relationships. Most practitioners conduct assessments to aid in making diagnostic determinations and treatment plans. Although most mental health professionals do not conduct polygraphs, real-world application for practitioners certainly consists of conducting a thorough evaluation, which includes psychological tests, clinical interviewing, behavioral observation, and a patient history. There are some instances in which practitioners do use polygraph data for criminal cases and for preemployment screening. (Iacono & Patrick, 2018).

Some psychological assessments gather information about the likelihood of lying in various ways. People may lie to look good (impression management), to look "crazy" or to have a psychological disorder, to minimize their pain or symptoms, to exaggerate their symptoms, to assume a sick role, or for some external gain. A comprehensive book on clinical assessment of malingering and deception has discussed the various assessments, their use, and research support (see Rogers & Bender, 2018). Thus, we do not present an exhaustive list of tests and assessments used for deception and malingering here.

One of the most commonly used clinical personality inventories is the Minnesota Multiphasic Personality Inventory—2 (MMPI-2; Butcher et al., 2001; Greene, 2011). The MMPI-2 contains validity scales and indexes that can indicate self-unfavorable or self-favorable reporting of psychopathology (Butcher et al., 2001; Greene, 2011). Similarly, the Personality Assessment Inventory (PAI) is another commonly used assessment, which some view as more straightforward or easily interpretable than the MMPI-2 (Greene, 2011; Morey, 1996). Comparable to the MMPI-2, it contains validity scales that indicate if a person may be trying to present a positive or negative impression (Greene, 2011; Morey, 1996). The Millon Clinical Multiaxial Inventory—IV (MCMI-IV) is another test that contains validity indices that can suggest underreporting of difficulties or whether a person might be "faking bad" (Greene, 2011; Millon et al., 2015). The Structured Interview of Reported Symptoms—2nd Edition (SIRS-2) is designed to assess intentional distortions or fabrications of self-reported symptoms (Rogers et al., 2010; Rogers & Bender, 2018).

ASSESSMENT OF PATHOLOGICAL LYING

The literature covering psychological assessments related to pathological lying is scant. Some early work references the general intellectual functioning of pathological liars. With the advent of standardized intelligence testing, others have examined aspects of intelligence and cognitive functioning as they relate to pathological lying. Our recent research extends into the area of providing data on the clinical and personality profiles of pathological liars.

Intelligence

Intelligence and its assessment has been another topic studied in conjunction with pathological lying. Healy and Healy (1915) were among the first to report on the intelligence of individuals who engaged in pathological lying. They discussed intelligence generally as good to excellent when discussing some case studies. However, at this time, intelligence testing was just starting to develop. Years later, B. H. King and Ford (1988) examined the intelligence of pathological liars. Their findings were of a bimodal grouping: one group with average to slightly below average intelligence and another group that had a superior intellect. B. H. King and Ford (1988) also reported that of eight cases, five displayed significantly better verbal ability (VIQ) compared with performance (PIQ). Some recent research has found that children who are good liars tend to perform better on verbal working memory tests (Alloway et al., 2015). Executive functioning related to working memory and inhibitory control play a role in children's ability to tell prosocial lies (Williams et al., 2016). The role of cognitive functioning in general is instrumental in understanding lying behavior (Leduc et al., 2017; Talwar & Crossman, 2011; Talwar et al., 2019).

Clinical and Personality Assessments

Adding to the limited assessment data of pathological lying, we recently conducted an assessment study (Curtis & Hart, 2021a). Our intent was to conduct clinical interviews and specific assessment procedures with people who identified as pathological liars. Much of what is presented in this section is technical and may be of interest only to people with expertise in administering psychological assessments. However, there is also much useful information that should be understandable to other professionals and the layperson.

We contacted people and asked if they or others have considered them to be a pathological liar or if they have told excessive lies. Participants were asked to complete the MMPI-2 (Butcher et al., 2001), the MCMI-IV (Millon et al., 2015), the Survey of Pathological Lying (SPL; Appendix A, this volume; Curtis & Hart, 2020), and the Distress Questionnaire—5 (DQ-5; Batterham et al., 2016). Also, we conducted semistructured interviews.

Findings from the SPL were that the average number of lies told within a 24-hour day was approximately 13. The greatest impairment in functioning was in social relationships. All participants indicated distress on the DQ-5 based on sensitivity cut points (≥ 11). Of the eight participants, five indicated that their lies put themselves or others in danger. Six of the eight participants indicated that they had never been formally diagnosed by a licensed mental health provider.

Regarding the MMPI-2 profiles, the major finding was an elevated Infrequency (F) and Back Infrequency (F_B) scales (see Table 7.1). Although elevated T scores on the F and F_B scales may be an invalid profile, it can also be due to a self-unfavorable report of psychopathology (Greene, 2011). Elevated scores on the F and F_B can represent severity of distress and a severe behavior disorder (Greene, 2011). Higher scores on the F scale have been found within clinical samples and state hospital inpatients, compared with MMPI-2 normative group (Greene, 2011). Given the relatively lower scores on the Infrequency Psychopathy (F_P) and the other validity indices,

Table 7.1

Minnesota Multiphasic Personality Inventory–2 Validity Scale Averages for a Pathological Lying Sample

	VRIN	TRIN	F	F_B	F_P	FBS	L	K	S
M	54.38	64.25	86.63	90.88	70.38	64.75	44.38	36.75	36.13
SD	11.76	10.25	23.35	16.80	20.74	15.24	5.93	6.80	6.58
Minimum	34	50	41	58	49	43	38	30	30
Maximum	70	80	120	120	113	90	52	47	49

Note. F = Infrequency scale; F_B = Back Infrequency scale; FBS = Fake Bad scale; F_P = Infrequency Psychopathy index; K = Defensiveness scale; L = Lie scale; S = Superlative Self-Preservation scale; TRIN = True Response Inconsistency scale; VRIN = Variable Response Inconsistency scale.

along with clinical interview data and scores on the DQ-5, it is likely that the current pathological lying sample represents a group who were exhibiting distress and profiles of a behavioral disorder—namely, pathological lying. Most MMPI-2 profiles demonstrated elevated F and F_B scores.

In analyzing the clinical scales of the MMPI-2, it is important to keep in mind that elevations of the validity scales share overlapping items with clinical scales. For example, for the F scale, 15 items overlap with Scale 8 (Schizophrenia; Sc), nine items overlap with Scale 6 (Paranoia; Pa), and four items overlap with Scale 4 (Psychopathic Deviate; Pd; Greene, 2011). Similarly, the F_B scale contains 10 items from Scale 8 and two items with Scale 6 and Scale 7 (Greene, 2011). From the collective clinical profile data, the highest elevation was Scale 8 (see Table 7.2). Scores between 65 and 89 on Sc are marked and indicate difficulties in logic, concentration, poor judgment, or a thought disorder (Greene, 2011). Additionally, elevated scores on Sc may represent feeling alienated, which could reflect situational or personal distress. Another marked elevation is Scale 6, which could indicate being suspicious, hostile, overly sensitive, and vocalization. Scale 7 also contained marked elevations, which could reflect being worried, tense, or indecisive (Greene, 2011). Last, Scale 2 showed marked elevations, which could indicate depressed mood about life or themselves, cognitions of guilt, and withdrawal or avoidance of social interactions (Greene, 2011).

Table 7.2

Minnesota Multiphasic Personality Inventory–2 Clinical Scale Averages for a Pathological Lying Sample

	Hs	D	Hy	Pd	MF	Pa	Pt	Sc	Ma	Si
M	67.25	72.38	58.50	67.25	56.25	76.63	74.50	80.88	62.63	64.00
SD	14.13	12.16	7.45	13.35	10.55	14.90	7.89	17.94	11.58	8.68
Minimum	51	55	47	49	38	56	61	53	47	49
Maximum	94	86	71	87	67	97	87	113	81	73

Note. D = Depression; Hs = Hypochondriasis; Hy = Hysteria; Ma = Mania; MF = Masculinity/Femininity; Pa = Paranoia; Pd = Psychopathic Deviate; Pt = Psychasthenia; Sc = Schizophrenia; Si = Social Introversion.

MCMI-IV profiles revealed that the pathological lying sample had elevated scores on the Disclosure and Debasement validity indices (see Table 7.3). High scores on Disclosure and Debasement can indicate fake bad profiles, or elevations could indicate a "cry for help" (Groth-Marnat & Wright, 2016, p. 433). Of the clinical personality patterns, the Melancholic (DFMelan) scale contained the highest elevation (80) in the group, although the clinical disorder range is often a base rate score of 85 or higher. This scale reflects dimensions of passive and pain and individuals may have thoughts of worthlessness, inadequacy, guilt, and self-criticism as well as reflecting an orientation toward the future being pessimistic (Groth-Marnat & Wright, 2016). Elevations were also observed in the Clinical Syndromes, specifically with Bipolar Spectrum (BIPspe) and Generalized Anxiety (GENanx). The elevated GENanx indicates complaints of apprehension, tension, or difficulties relaxing (Groth-Marnat & Wright, 2016). Groth-Marnat and Wright (2016) also discussed that the anxiety can be specifically focused to social situations. Thus, the participants' elevated scores on GENanx could reflect exaggerations or could be related to the anxiety felt following telling lies to others. The elevated BIPspe scores are indicative of mood swings (being elated or depressed) and may reflect a tendency toward impulsiveness (Groth-Marnat & Wright, 2016). Similarly, the collective elevated scores could reflect exaggerations of mood or impulsivity or could reveal some of the features of pathological lying as being impulsive and the shifting of moods based on telling a lie in the moment to remorse felt after lying.

Let us now consider each individual and their assessment data. Participant 1 indicated that lying does not occur as frequently as it did in the past. The participant indicated that many lies told were themed around hiding a romantic relationship from parents. The participant's MMPI-2 profile fell largely within the normative range for validity indices and clinical scales (see Figure 7.1). In a clinical interview, the participant did not endorse diagnostic criteria for antisocial personality disorder. Regarding the MCMI-IV profile, the participant indicated a need for social approval based on a higher desirability score and a possible deficit in self-knowledge.

Participant 2 indicated that lying often resulted in impairment in social and occupational functioning. The participant indicated telling lies

Table 7.3

Millon Clinical Multiaxial Inventory–IV Base Rate Averages for a Pathological Lying Sample

	Base rate mean	SD	Min	Max
Validity				
Disclosure	78.25	14.95	43	92
Desirability	49.75	14.36	30	75
Debasement	76.25	17.81	38	93
Clinical personality patterns				
AASchd	66.50	23.97	9	80
SRAvoid	77.00	25.52	17	99
DFMelan	80.00	20.06	37	100
DADepn	71.50	11.53	50	90
SPHistr	41.88	15.62	26	72
EETurbu	50.13	19.98	18	75
CENarc	55.38	18.58	24	80
ADAntis	72.50	10.92	60	90
ADSadis	63.25	14.58	30	78
RCComp	50.38	9.47	33	63
DRNegat	67.00	28.05	0	87
AAMasoc	72.88	22.64	24	97
Severe personality pathology				
ESSchizoph	69.88	14.55	36	81
UBCycloph	71.00	29.92	0	96
MPParaph	66.25	27.35	0	84
Clinical syndromes				
GENanx	83.50	22.83	30	105
SOMsym	58.25	30.93	0	84
BIPspe	87.38	14.07	66	105
PERdep	78.50	24.49	20	96
ALCuse	74.00	13.65	59	95
DRGuse	67.50	31.83	0	103
P-Tstr	65.50	27.82	0	89

(continues)

Table 7.3

Millon Clinical Multiaxial Inventory–IV Base Rate Averages for a Pathological Lying Sample (*Continued*)

	Base rate mean	SD	Min	Max
	Severe Clinical Syndromes			
SCHspe	66.13	17.40	25	82
MAJdep	80.00	33.57	0	105
DELdis	60.63	25.04	0	78

Note. AAMasoc = Masochistic; AASchd = Schizoid; ADAntis = Antisocial; ADSadis = Sadistic; ALCuse = Alcohol Use; BIPspe = Bipolar Spectrum; CENarc = Narcissistic; DADepn = Dependent; DELdis = Delusional; DFMelan = Melancholic; DRGuse = Drug Use; DRNegat = Negativistic; EETurbu = Turbulent; ESSchizoph = Schizotypal; GENanx = Generalized Anxiety; MAJdep = Major Depression; Max = maximum; Min = minimum; MPParaph = Paranoid; PERdep = Persistent Depression; P-Tstr = Post-Traumatic Stress; RCComp = Compulsive; SCHspe = Schizophrenic Spectrum; SOMsym = Somatic Symptom; SPHistr = Histrionic; SRAvoid = Avoidant; UBCycloph = Borderline.

largely for impression management: to win people over, get friendships, have people offer help, and seek occupational promotions. However, the participant also mentioned that there would be times of lying just to lie and without a specific motivation in mind. Participant 2 stated that telling lies frequently led to positive consequences, where the situations seemed to be better and the person felt good telling the lie. Negative consequences from lying were often the loss of friendships. The participant discussed one lie told to a friend about where the participant was from. As time passed, along with interactions with the friend, the lie continued to grow, and the person said additional details were added. Participant 2's MMPI-2 profile displayed the elevated F, F_B, F_P, and Fake Bad (FBS) scales. The Inconsistency scales and the Lie (L), Defensiveness (K), and Superlative Self-Preservation (S) scales were within the normative or low range. The clinical profile revealed an 8–6–1 configuration (see Figure 7.2). Participant 2 discussed remorse for lying and reported having no legal problems. The participant's MCMI-IV results indicated that there may have been overreporting of actual symptoms and potentially exaggerated clinical syndrome scales.

Participant 3 reported that "I know my lying is toxic and I am trying to get help." The participant indicated telling numerous lies to friends,

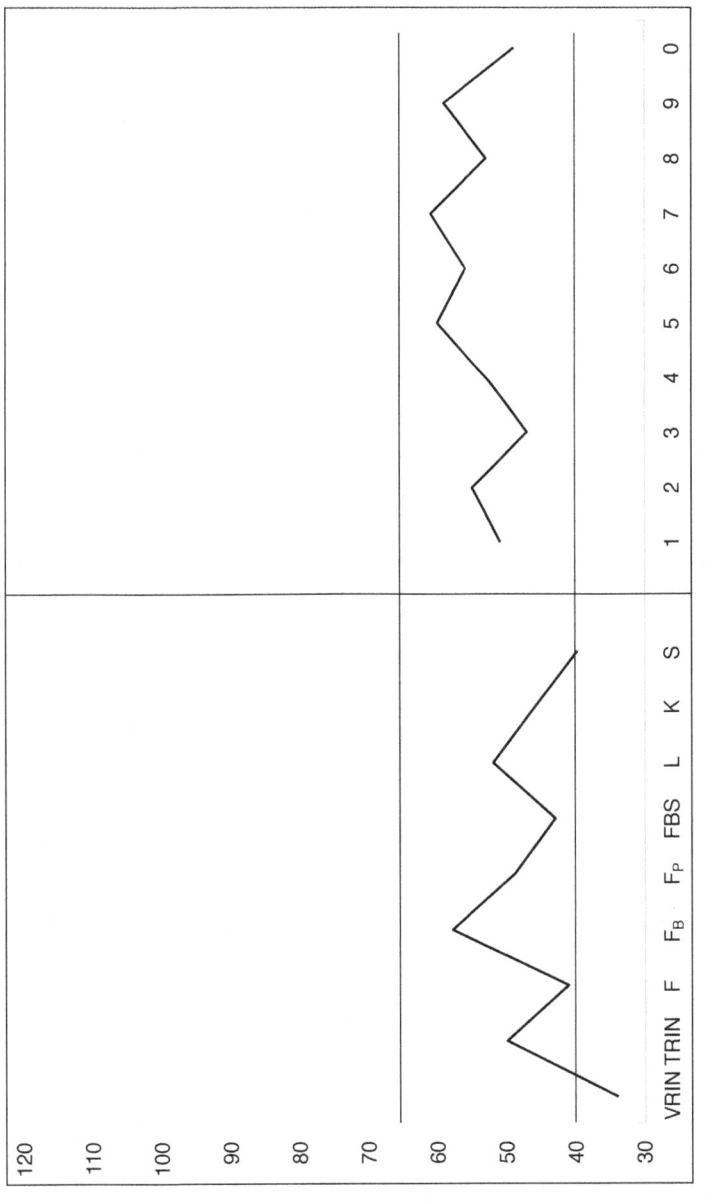

Figure 7.1

Participant 1 profile. F = Infrequency scale; F_B = Back Infrequency scale; FBS = Fake Bad scale; F_P = Infrequency Psychopathy index; K = Defensiveness scale; L = Lie scale; S = Superlative Self-Preservation scale; TRIN = True Response Inconsistency scale; VRIN = Variable Response Inconsistency scale.

PATHOLOGICAL LYING

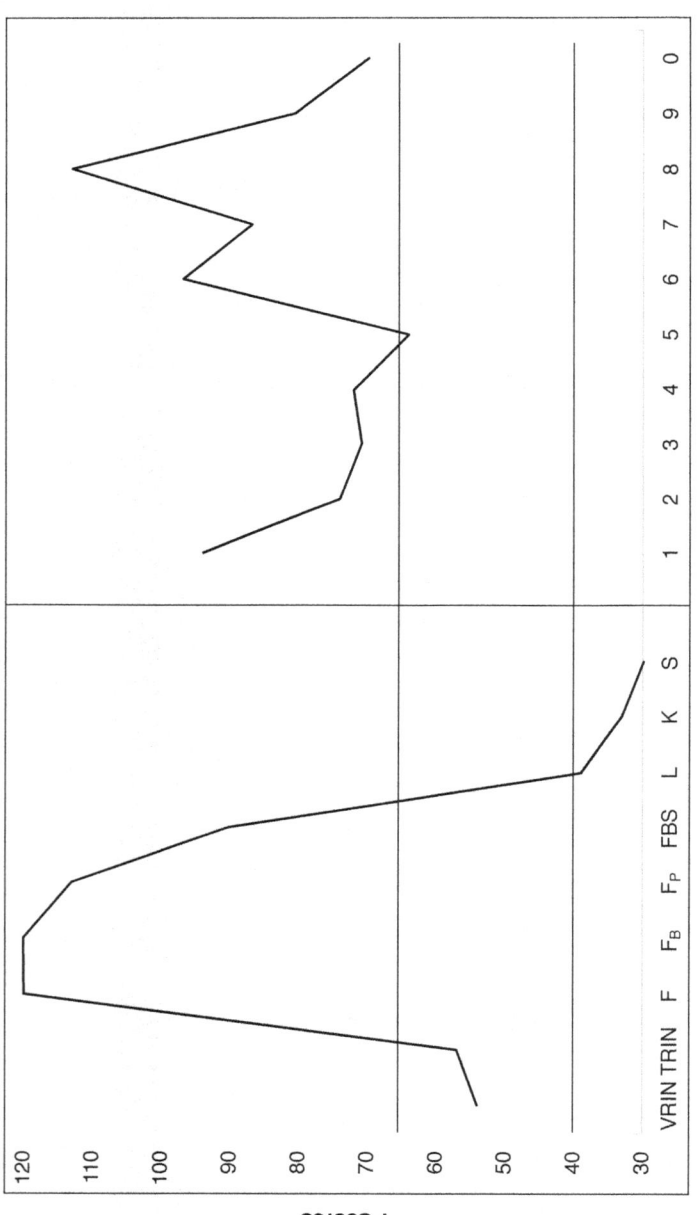

Figure 7.2

Participant 2 profile. F = Infrequency scale; F_B = Back Infrequency scale; FBS = Fake Bad scale; F_P = Infrequency Psychopathy index; K = Defensiveness scale; L = Lie scale; S = Superlative Self-Preservation scale; TRIN = True Response Inconsistency scale; VRIN = Variable Response Inconsistency scale.

148

in intimate relationships, to parents, and to get out of work. The partici-pant reported telling lies to appear better to others. Participant 3 discussed experiencing a mix of relief and anxiety when lying, sometimes feeling relief after telling a lie and other times feeling guilty and remorseful for lying. The participant indicated impulsivity in telling lies by stating that "my mouth is faster than my mind." In the clinical interview, the partici-pant did not meet diagnostic criteria for antisocial personality disorder. The participant reported no problems conforming to social norms and following the law, stated a deep regard for the well-being of others, was able to maintain a job, and often displayed remorse after lying or hurting others. A negative consequence from lying was often the loss of friend-ships. The participant discussed one lie told to a friend about where the participant was from. As time passed, along with interactions with the friend, the lie continued to grow, and the person said additional details were added. Participant 3's MMPI-2 profile displayed the elevated F and F_B, but other validity scales fell within the normative range. Clinical scales revealed a 4–6–8 profile (see Figure 7.3). The participant's responses on the MCMI-IV revealed a high level of disclosure and debasement, which may represent exaggerated symptoms or over-reporting of actual symptoms.

Participant 4 reported telling a lot of white lies, minimizing self, and trying to help others or make others feel better. The participant indicated lying less now than in the past. The participant reported being called a pathological liar by both parents. Participant 4's MMPI-2 profile displayed the elevated F and F_B, but other validity scales fell within the normative range (see Figure 7.4). The clinical profile revealed a spike on Scales 8 and 2. The participant's responses on the MCMI-IV revealed that there may be a tendency to magnify experiences of illness or to be self-pitying, or there may be feelings of vulnerability related to acute distress. The profile indi-cated that scores on the Clinical Syndrome may be exaggerated.

Participant 5 reported telling excessive lies often to protect others' feel-ings or to avoid being in a bad social situation. The participant reported that lies impaired relationships because people would often discover the lies, leading to the participant feeling guilty and others having less trust. Participant 5 reported feeling relief after telling a lie if others believed it

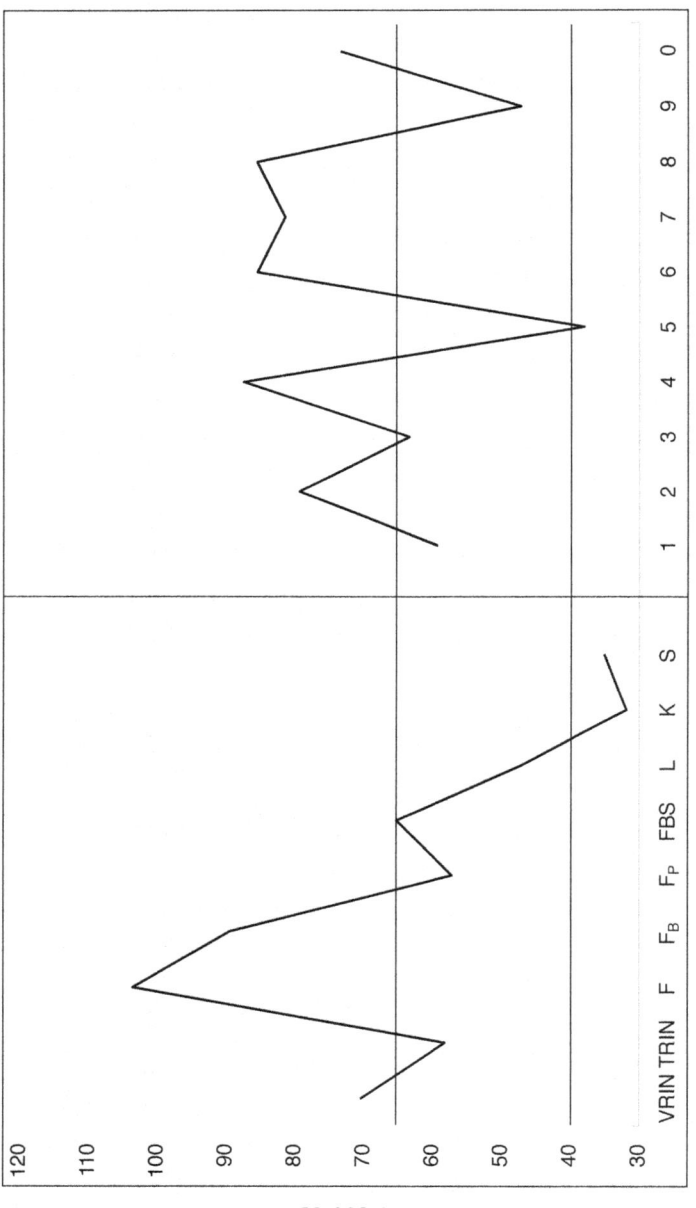

Figure 7.3

Participant 3 profile. F = Infrequency scale; F_B = Back Infrequency scale; FBS = Fake Bad scale; F_P = Infrequency Psychopathy index; K = Defensiveness scale; L = Lie scale; S = Superlative Self-Preservation scale; TRIN = True Response Inconsistency scale; VRIN = Variable Response Inconsistency scale.

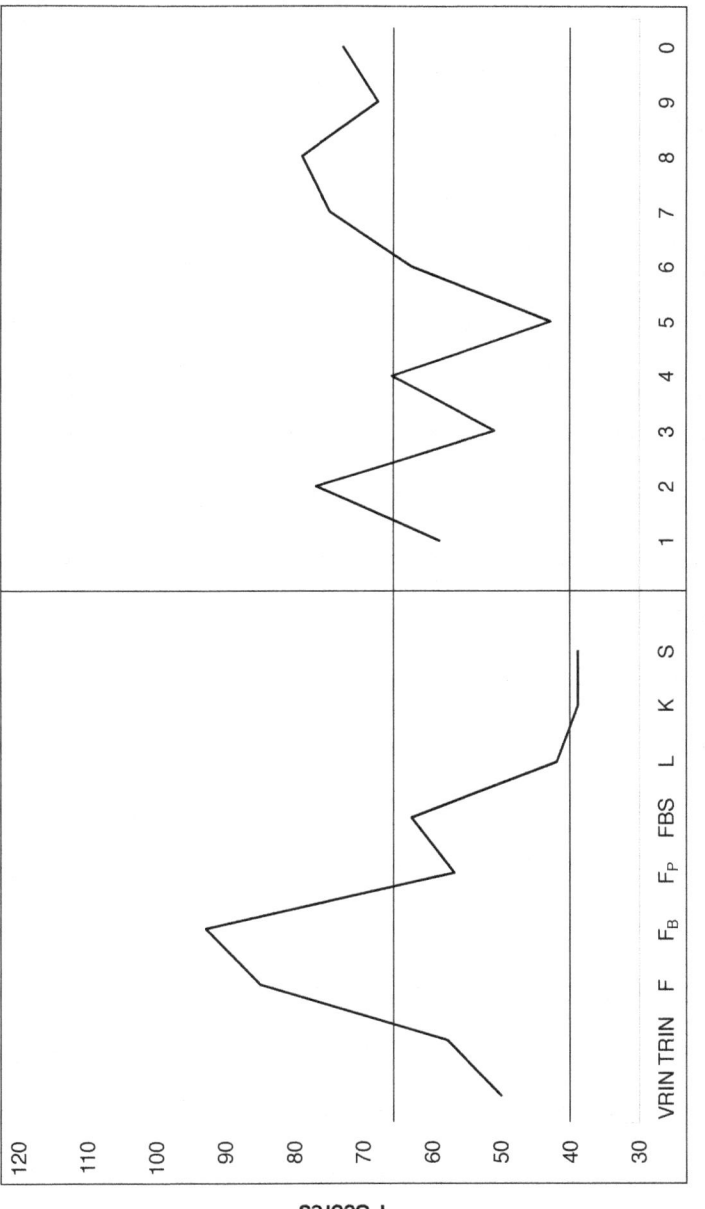

Figure 7.4

Participant 4 profile. F = Infrequency scale; F_B = Back Infrequency scale; FBS = Fake Bad scale; F_P = Infrequency Psychopathy index; K = Defensiveness scale; L = Lie scale; S = Superlative Self-Preservation scale; TRIN = True Response Inconsistency scale; VRIN = Variable Response Inconsistency scale.

but would feel guilty and remorseful if they discovered the deceptions. The participant stated feeling like "I have to lie" and "I shouldn't feel like I should lie." The participant did not meet diagnostic criteria for antisocial personality disorder. The participant reported no legal involvement or trouble, conformed to social norms, reported no aggression, and would often feel remorse when lies were discovered. Participant 5's MMPI-2 profile revealed some elevations with inconsistency scales (e.g., True Response Inconsistency [TRIN]) and elevated F, F_B, F_P, and FBS scales. The L, K, and S scales were within the normative or low range (see Figure 7.5). The clinical profile revealed a 2–4–7. Regarding the MCMI-IV profile, the participant indicated low self-confidence and problems with school and work. This participant's scores did not reveal elevated Debasement or very high Disclosure scores. The participant's highest elevations were on the Melancholic scale (DFMelan) and Major Depression scale (MAJdep).

Participant 6 reported telling numerous "successful lies" and not ever having them detected by others. The participant indicated lying now just as much as ever and that the lies often affected social relationships and finances. The participant said, "I know it's wrong but don't know why I do it" and reported that lies tended to grow bigger from initial smaller lies. The participant discussed a lie that began in school and grew, lying to parents, and then lying to a psychotherapist for years. The participant did not meet diagnostic criteria for antisocial personality disorder. The participant indicated following the rules, not having legal problems, feeling remorse for actions, no aggression toward others, and no concerns with irresponsibility. Participant 6's MMPI-2 profile revealed elevated F, F_B, and F_P scales. The Variable Response Inconsistency (VRIN), TRIN, FBS, L, K, and S scales were within the normative range (see Figure 7.6). The clinical profile revealed a 6–8–2. The participant's responses on the MCMI-IV revealed an elevated Disclosure score, which may be related to over reporting. The participant indicated problems with loneliness, alienation, and thoughts of worthlessness.

Participant 7 reported telling numerous lies in high school, which often affected relationships and finances. The participant stated that the biggest lie told was to parents, telling them that the participant was not

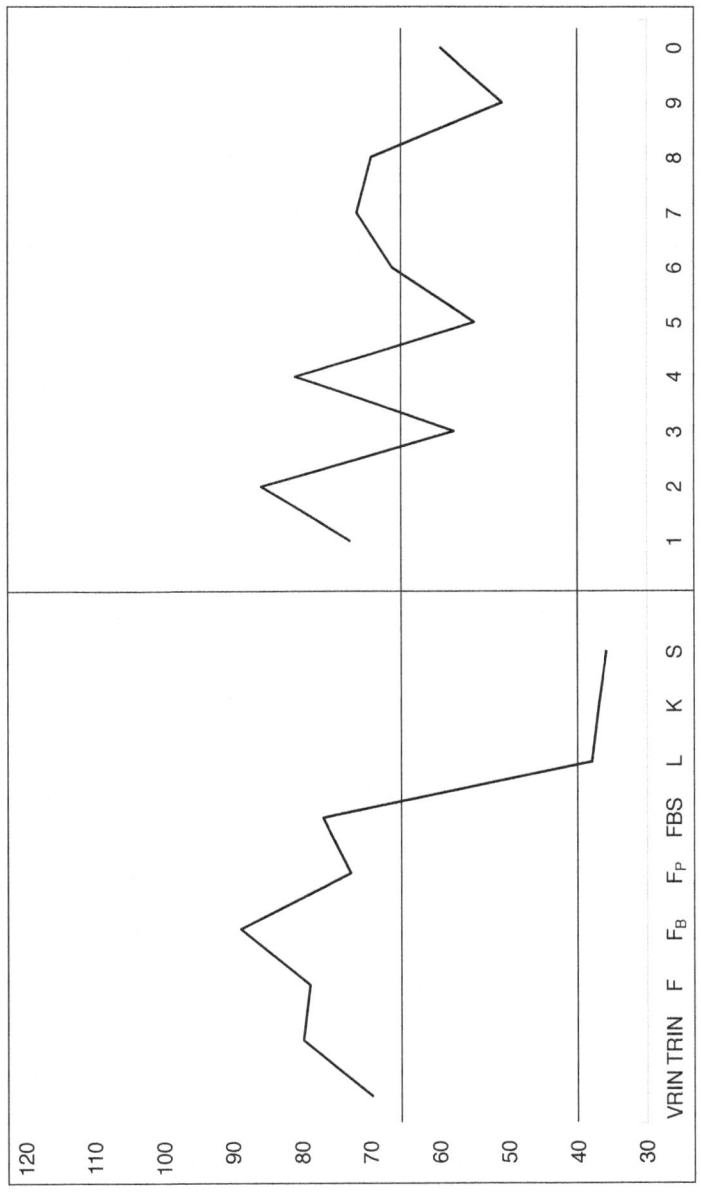

Figure 7.5

Participant 5 profile. F = Infrequency scale; F_B = Back Infrequency scale; FBS = Fake Bad scale; F_P = Infrequency Psychopathy index; K = Defensiveness scale; L = Lie scale; S = Superlative Self-Preservation scale; TRIN = True Response Inconsistency scale; VRIN = Variable Response Inconsistency scale.

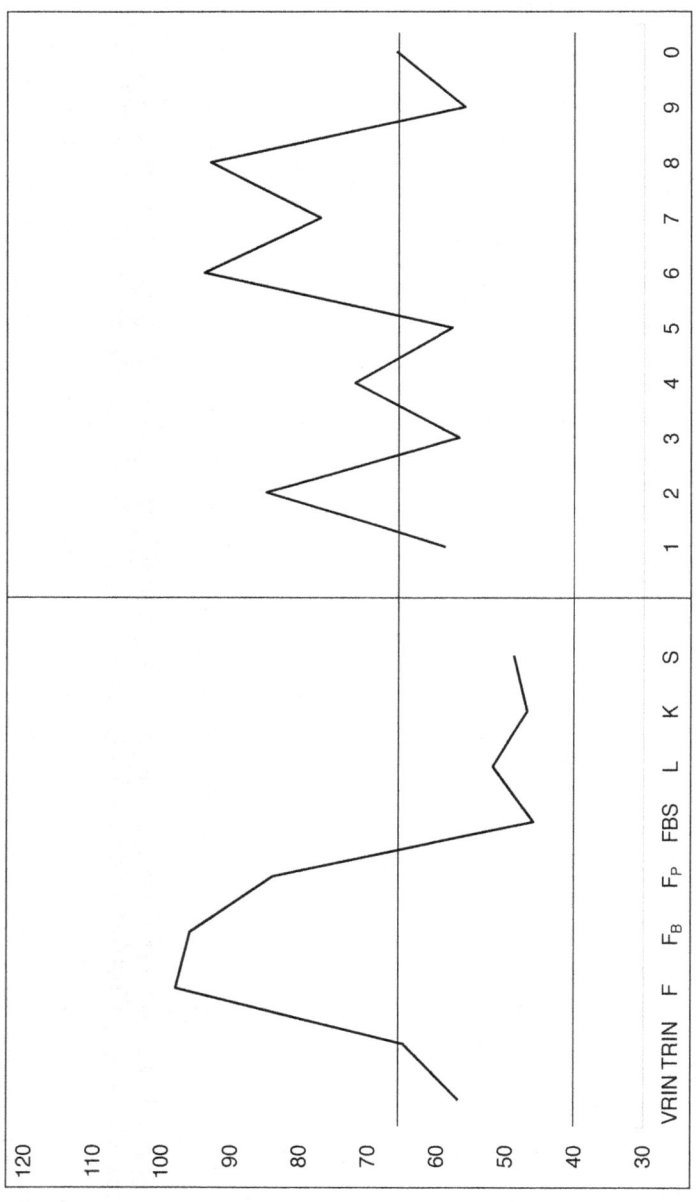

Figure 7.6

Participant 6 profile. F = Infrequency scale; F_B = Back Infrequency scale; FBS = Fake Bad scale; F_P = Infrequency Psychopathy index; K = Defensiveness scale; L = Lie scale; S = Superlative Self-Preservation scale; TRIN = True Response Inconsistency scale; VRIN = Variable Response Inconsistency scale.

high from a substance when they were. The participant indicated lying for no reason sometimes and other times lied to avoid disappointing others or to secretly maintain an intimate relationship. The participant did not meet diagnostic criteria for antisocial personality disorder. The participant denied legal problems, denied impulsivity or failures to plan, indicated remorse, and displayed consistent responsibility with occupations and academic coursework. Participant 7's MMPI-2 profile revealed elevated TRIN, F, and F_B scales. Other validity indices were within the normative range. The clinical elevation was on Scale 8 (see Figure 7.7). The participant's MCMI-IV profile revealed elevated Disclosure and Debasement scores. The participant either has a tendency to exaggerate experienced illness or is feeling vulnerable with acute distress.

Participant 8 reported that lies told had negatively affected relationships and finances. The participant indicated that lies were sometimes told to gain friendships. Discovered deceptions often led to the loss of friendships. The participant indicated that telling lies initially felt good and safe but later resulted in feeling guilt. The participant indicated that lies often grew from an initial lie—for example, lying about having a migraine— and subsequently exaggerating symptoms and features. The participant indicated other psychopathology, having been formally diagnosed with bipolar disorder and generalized anxiety disorder by a licensed mental health practitioner. In the clinical interview, the patient did not endorse symptoms that represented antisocial personality disorder. The participant's MMPI-2 profile revealed elevated TRIN, F, F_B, and F_P scales. Other validity indices were within the normative range. The clinical elevation was a 1–6 (see Figure 7.8). The participant's MCMI-IV profile revealed elevated Disclosure and Debasement scores. Similar to other profiles, the participant may have a tendency to magnify the experience of illness or is feeling vulnerable based on acute distress.

The assessment data add another dimension to understanding pathological lying. Namely, there were key features that seemed to emerge, even though the data consisted of a low sample size. With the exception of the first participant, who had a normal profile, the assessment responses seemed to consistently reflect a pattern of over-reporting of symptoms or symptom severity. Thus, overreporting could be due to lying through

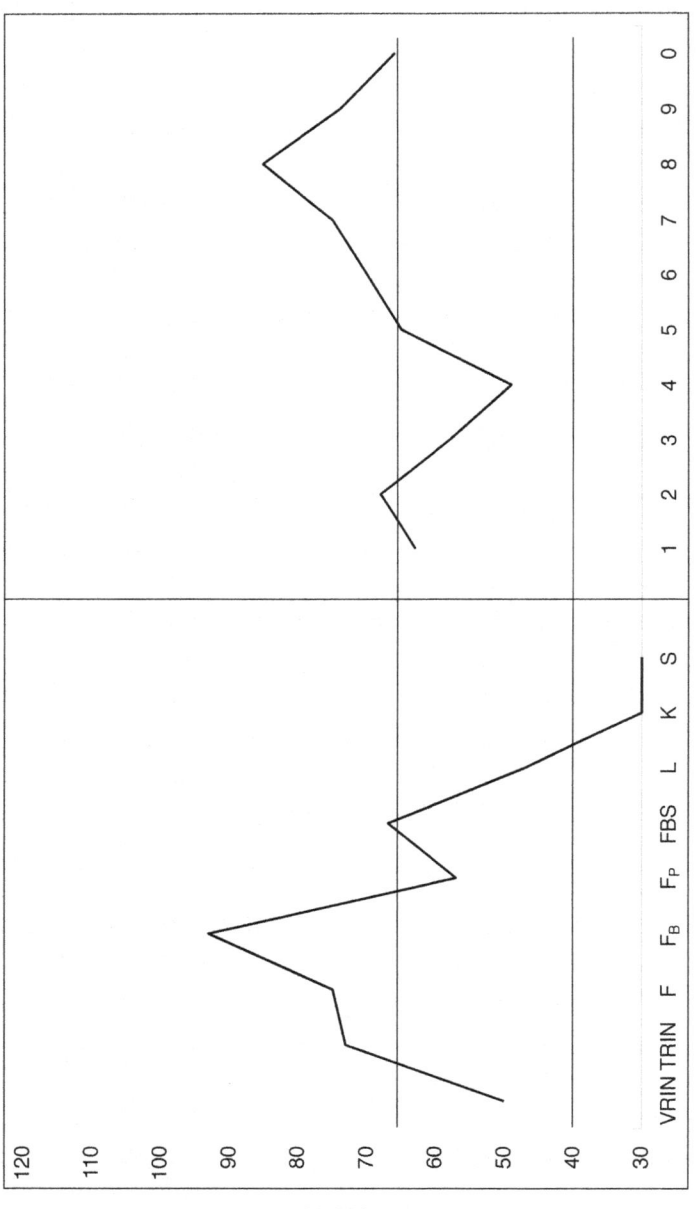

Figure 7.7

Participant 7 profile. F = Infrequency scale; F_B = Back Infrequency scale; FBS = Fake Bad scale; F_P = Infrequency Psychopathy index; K = Defensiveness scale; L = Lie scale; S = Superlative Self-Preservation scale; TRIN = True Response Inconsistency scale; VRIN = Variable Response Inconsistency scale.

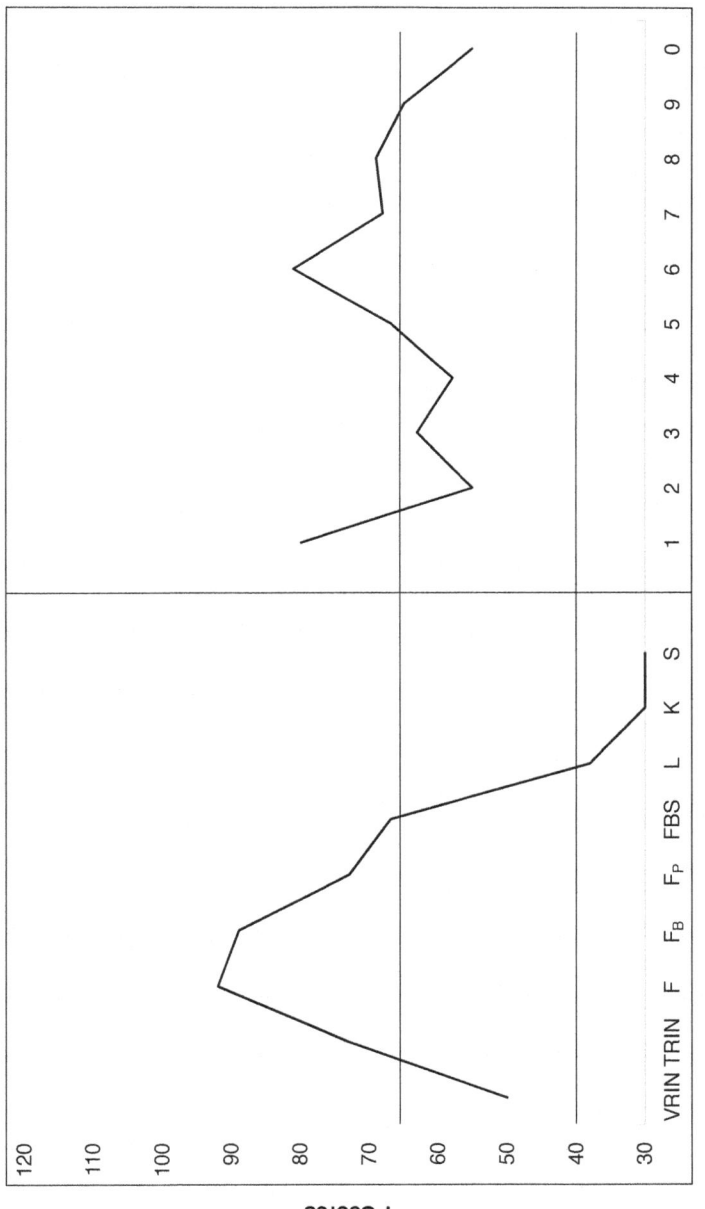

Scales

Figure 7.8

Participant 8 profile. F = Infrequency scale; F_B = Back Infrequency scale; FBS = Fake Bad scale; F_P = Infrequency Psychopathy index; K = Defensiveness scale; L = Lie scale; S = Superlative Self-Preservation scale; TRIN = True Response Inconsistency scale; VRIN = Variable Response Inconsistency scale.

exaggeration of symptoms. However, the responses could represent distress from symptoms, specifically those related to pathological lying. Given that all participants indicated general psychological distress on the DQ-5 and reports of their excessive lying causing them distress in the clinical interview, it stands to reason that responses on MMPI-2 and MCMI-IV may represent symptom severity. Last, another possibility is that both are true, in that the sample exaggerated symptoms and actually experienced severe distress from symptoms.

These data should provide clinicians and researchers with assessment data that reflect pathological lying. However, the data are limited by the small sample size, and generalizability should be done with caution. The assessment data and scales can be used to help clinicians make diagnostic determinations about patients who may engage in pathological lying. These data can be used in conjunction with a clinical interview and diagnostic criteria to help determine a diagnosis.

Although the clinical profiles from standardized and psychometrically established assessments will aid in the understanding of pathological lying, there has yet to be an assessment specifically designed for pathological lying. Not having a specific psychological test for pathological lying was a concern of Dike and colleagues (2005). In Chapter 5, we introduced our measure to examine and classify pathological lying (Curtis & Hart, 2020b). Recently, we used our proposed definition of pathological lying to develop the Pathological Lying Inventory (PLI), which is a 33-item measure that contains six factors (see Appendix B, this volume; Hart, Curtis, & Randell, 2022). Through two studies, we found the PLI to be a valid measure that demonstrated high reliability. We hope this instrument will also be useful for practitioners to assess and for researchers to classify pathological lying. Future research may examine the predictive validity of the assessment profiles and PLI to accurately classify pathological lying.

THE ASSESSMENT PROCESS

The utility of assessments is providing a clinician with data about the individual, collectively, to aid in decision making or diagnostic determinations. We have presented assessment data that may inform practitioners about various response styles and clinical profiles on some standardized psychological tests. A formal diagnostic entity provides the benefits of classification, which includes research and ultimately treatment of the individual. The downside is that the assessments typically gather information about the individual's propensity to lie or response style and do not tell a clinician if and when the person may be lying in the moment. These data would require lie-detection ability or a confession from the patient.

8

Diagnosis

Think of the auto mechanic who indicates that your car has a torn engine belt that needs to be replaced. Think of the physician who discovers a person has a broken leg bone. Do these thought experiments elicit thoughts of resolve to discover the problem, or do they lead to thinking that mechanics and physicians are pathologizing people and vehicles? The mental health field is viewed differently in regard to provisions of diagnosis, where there is a public perception of caution and concern that diagnosis is used to stimulate growth in the medicinal marketplace (Curtis & Kelley, 2021). To reiterate from Chapter 5, a diagnosis is not a nasty epithet but is merely a name or label for a set of symptoms that typically cluster together.

Assessments are used to aid in making diagnostic determinations, which, in turn, lead to treatments. For example, when a person goes to the emergency department and has an X-ray of their leg (assessment) and

https://doi.org/10.1037/0000305-008
Pathological Lying: Theory, Research, and Practice, by D. A. Curtis and C. L. Hart

learns that they have a broken leg (diagnosis), then this diagnosis is a label to describe the symptoms (pain, difficulty with movement, etc.) that someone has resultant of their condition—a broken leg. Following the diagnosis, a cast and pain medication (treatment) may be prescribed.

The *Diagnostic and Statistical Manual of Mental Disorders* (5th ed.; *DSM-5*; American Psychiatric Association, 2013) indicates that reliable diagnoses are crucial to guide treatments, identify prevalence, identify and classify groups for clinical research, and record public health information. Thus, diagnosis is a crucial step for treatment and has benefits for other domains. When there is no name or label, then what is done? There are two possible outcomes when a diagnosis does not exist: the person's disorder goes unrecognized or the person receives another diagnosis.

For pathological lying, the lack of a diagnostic entity has resulted in these consequences. Although it may be unclear how often it has gone unrecognized, we discuss some of our recent research findings that indicate practitioners can reliably diagnose pathological lying. We also discuss the consequences of not having a formal diagnostic category.

PSYCHOTHERAPISTS' EXPERIENCES AND ABILITY TO DIAGNOSE

In a study we conducted (Curtis & Hart, 2021c) with psychologists and other mental health practitioners, we provided them with our definition of pathological lying and asked them to determine whether four cases met diagnostic criteria for pathological lying. Two of the cases were vignettes of pathological lying (one from Thom et al., 2017, and one we created). Another case was a person with antisocial personality disorder (ASPD; from Covrig et al., 2013). The last case was a person who had trichotillomania (from Curtis & Kelley, 2020a), which is a psychological disorder that consists of repeated hair-pulling behavior or frequent urges to pull one's hair. After each case study, we asked practitioners whether the person met diagnostic criteria for pathological lying and whether there were any additional diagnoses considered for the person. If they believed that the person did not meet diagnostic criteria for pathological lying, then we asked them what diagnosis would be appropriate.

Of the practitioners who had worked with a patient who engaged in pathological lying, a majority (68%) provided the patient with a diagnosis (Curtis & Hart, 2021c). Although clinicians provided a variety of diagnoses (see Appendix C, this volume), more than half (56%) of the participants indicated that they diagnosed the patient with some personality disorder (see Figure 8.1). The most common personality disorder diagnosis was ASPD (16%), followed by a general personality disorder or a mix of personality disorders (15%), borderline personality disorder (13%), and narcissistic personality disorder (5%).

It could be that the consequences of pathological lying not being regarded as a diagnostic entity led some practitioners to offer a diagnosis, albeit the wrong one. Practitioners, who presumably were motivated to help, may have merely been doing the best they could with the limited diagnostic options available. A limited tool may influence a clinician to work with what they have, providing a diagnosis that is most similar in nature to what is being observed, even if not an ideal fit. It is somewhat intuitive that practitioners would consider ASPD as a diagnosis when a

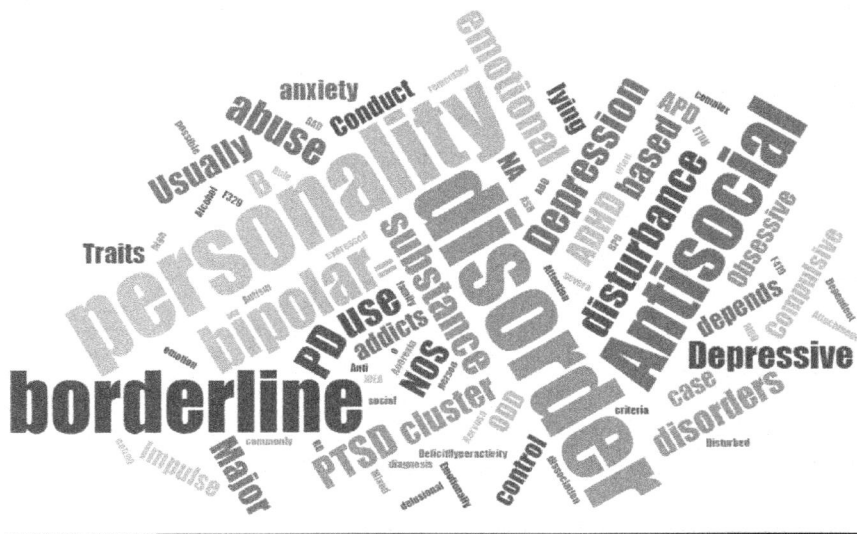

Figure 8.1

Word cloud of diagnoses provided for pathological lying. Data from Curtis and Hart (2021c).

patient presents with pathological lying as their concern. One of the diagnostic criteria for ASPD is deceitfulness. However, we discuss later how these two are distinct and can be differentiated.

As you may recall from Chapter 6, one anonymous person in our blog study indicated that they were incorrectly diagnosed with ASPD, resulting in not wanting to go back to a clinician (Curtis & Hart, 2021b). The person stated, "I'm a textbook pathological liar. . . . But I would like help with this, any tips? . . . I got falsely diagnosed with AsPD not long ago, so I refuse to go back." At least in this case, an incorrect diagnosis of a personality disorder demotivated the individual to seek out psychological services.

Approximately 32% of practitioners in our study did not provide a diagnosis. The good news here is that patients were not incorrectly classified. The potential downside was that patients who engaged in pathological lying were perhaps not provided treatment for pathological lying. However, we did not specifically assess this within our study.

Our findings did present a silver lining. Of the 156 practitioners who read the four vignettes, most (86%) were able to correctly discern the pathological lying vignettes from the other two (ASPD and trichotillomania). The ability to correctly classify was not associated with educational degree, type of license, or years of experience. These data indicate that practitioners can discern pathological lying from other psychological disorders, and we could infer that, had pathological lying been available as a diagnosis, it might have been applied in a number of cases.

DIAGNOSTIC FRAMEWORK FOR PATHOLOGICAL LYING

To remedy the concern of a limited diagnostic toolbox or of practitioners providing another diagnosis for pathological lying, we suggest a diagnostic framework based on past clinical cases, existing literature, our definition, a theoretical model, and research. Our definition can be used to easily map onto major nosological systems and provide parameters for clinical assessment. We discuss a framework for pathological lying as a diagnostic entity, its structure, and differential diagnoses. For the *DSM-5*, we propose that pathological lying would fit categorically under Obsessive-Compulsive and Related Disorders or under Disruptive, Impulse-Control, and Conduct Disorders (American Psychiatric Association, 2013). For the *International Classification of Diseases* (World Health Organization, 1992), pathological lying could fit under disorders of social functioning with onset specific to childhood and adolescence or under impulse disorders (F63). The framework we suggest for pathological lying diagnostic criteria is as follows:

a. A persistent and pervasive pattern of excessive lying behavior occurring for longer than 6 months.
b. The symptoms cause clinically significant impairment in social, occupational, or other areas of functioning and cause clinically significant distress.
c. The behavior is not attributable to the physiological effects of a substance or to another medical condition.
d. The disturbance is not better explained by the symptoms of another mental disorder (e.g., antisocial personality disorder; psychopathy; delusional disorder or another psychotic disorder).

Specify if:

Primary: Excessive lying with a variety of topics.
Secondary: Conditions that are associated with pathological lying or where lying has a focused theme or content (e.g., factitious disorder).

Specify if:

Pseudologia fantastica: The lies told consist of extremely exaggerated stories or life details that appear fantastical or not rooted in reality.

The primary and secondary specifiers would allow for more specificity in diagnosis and provide specific research markers. These specifiers were suggested by Dike and colleagues (2005) and credited to Healy and Healy (1915). They suggested a classification structure of pathological lying that consists of primary and secondary pathological lying. They proposed primary pathological lying as an independent diagnostic entity and secondary pathological lying to include various conditions that are associated with pathological lying. Dike (2020) made the case that pathological lying is a distinct disorder and can be viewed as a superordinate category. Thus, secondary pathological lying could consist of narrower subcategories of pathological lying, where there is a condition that includes excessive lying in a specific area or theme, such as factitious disorder (Dike, 2020).

Pathological lying could consist of meeting diagnostic criteria with or without factitious disorder. "A review of the literature reveals a subgroup of individuals who exhibited pathological lying but without evidence of Factitious Disorder or any other overt psychiatric disorder" (Dike et al., 2005, p. 346). There are published cases of individuals who were diagnosed with factitious disorder and pseudologia fantastica (pathological lying; e.g., Melin et al., 2008). Many, but not all, case studies of pathological lying involve factitious disorder–like symptoms, yet the people also lie in many other realms. Thus, factitious disorder can be viewed as a narrower category, where lies are specifically focused on symptoms, often motivated to assume a sick role. Factitious disorder was originally referred to as Munchausen's syndrome, coined by Asher in 1951. The *DSM-5* indicates that criteria for factitious disorder includes "Falsification of physical or psychological signs or symptoms, or induction of injury or disease, associated with identified deception" and "the deceptive behavior is evident even in the absence of obvious external rewards" (American Psychiatric Association, 2013, p. 324). Deception is a key feature of factitious disorder, though the theme is specific to physical or psychological symptoms. Even if one were to actually induce injury, disease, or symptoms instead of falsifying symptoms, the actions are "associated with deception" (American Psychiatric Association, 2013, p. 324). The individuals who induce illness or injury are deceptive by lying via omission, not telling others what they have done to assume a sick role.

Along with Dike's (2020) suggestion for primary and secondary specifiers, we recommend another specifier: *pseudologia fantastica*. Pseudologia fantastica has been referenced in case studies and literature to encompass two aspects of pathological lying. In one instance, people have used the term to reference pathological lying, as we have defined it, often telling numerous lies that impair social relationships and cause marked distress. On the other hand, there are instances where the lies are truly fantastic, or heavily exaggerated. Clinical case studies indicate that in a smaller percentage of people who tell excessive lies, their lies have distinctive features—namely, exaggerated stories or life details that appear implausible, fantastic, and not rooted in reality. Ford (1996) also discussed pseudologia fantastica in this manner. Thus, those who tell excessive lies that are themed around implausible or impossible details may be described as exhibiting symptoms of pathological lying/pseudologia fantastica.

DIFFERENTIAL DIAGNOSIS

One of the arguments that likely contributed to pathological lying not being recognized as a diagnostic entity was that it was not viewed as an entirely distinct psychological disorder. Some authors suggested that pathological lying should be viewed as a symptom of other psychological disorders, such as narcissistic personality disorder or factitious disorder (Garlipp, 2017; Newmark et al., 1999). Others have argued that pathological lying can be considered a psychological disorder but that it is often comorbid with personality disorders (Muzinic et al., 2016). However, we tend to agree with Healy and Healy (1915), who suggested that pathological lying is distinct and occurs in the absence of other psychological disorders. We present various other psychological disorders and show how they can be distinguished from pathological lying.

Delusional Disorder, Schizophrenia, or Other Psychotic Disorder

At first glance, it may be easy to say that someone who speaks an untruth is a liar. However, it is crucial to recall the definition of lying. Lying involves an intentional and deliberate attempt by a person to try to make someone else believe something that they do not believe to be true. If a person were delusional, then they would be speaking about untrue beliefs that they actually believe to be true. Therefore, a person who was delusional would not be lying. For example, consider a person who believes that the FBI has been bugging their house, car, and workplace in an attempt to arrest them, when in fact there are no bugs or attempts from the FBI (a delusion of persecution). If this person tells others that the FBI has been secretly listening to their conversations, they would not be lying because they believe the message that they are communicating to others. Although the information is untrue, the communication is not a deception. Thus, it is highly important to clarify whether a person truly believes what they are saying or whether they are delusional. Thus, if a person meets diagnostic criteria for a delusional disorder or other psychotic disorder (e.g., schizophrenia, schizoaffective disorder), then clarifying their actual belief is crucial. To consider pathological lying with a delusional disorder or other psychotic disorder, it would be imperative not only to establish whether the individual believes the untrue statements but also whether the lying behavior occurs in the absence of delusions or psychotic episodes.

One anonymous person from our blog study who self-identified as a compulsive liar explicitly indicated that lying was not due to a delusion:

> I am a compulsive liar. I am not psychotic or delusional, I recognize that what I say is not honest. I don't understand why I do this—I can even hear myself doing it—and I internally scream "STOP" but I keep going. I do not lie to gain control, I do not lie because I enjoy it. It does not feel good to lie. I do lie to make myself seem more positive. I lie to make other people happy.

Discerning whether a person actually believes their untrue statements can be much more challenging.

Malingering

Malingering (*DSM-5* V65.2; American Psychiatric Association, 2013) is a specific clinical condition that is based on lying specifically for some external incentives or gains. "Malingerers lie; therefore, liars malinger" is a faulty and illogical claim that often leads people to believe the faulty conclusion that deception is evidence of malingering (Rogers, 2018). Not all liars are malingering. Further, not all pathological liars are malingerers. In fact, Rogers (2018) indicated that base rates for malingering vary, largely dependent on the "referral question and individual circumstances" (p. 9). Pathological lying is a consistent and pervasive pattern of lying. People who engage in pathological lying often are not motivated to lie for a specific external gain. In fact, most pathological liars indicated lying for no reason (Curtis & Hart, 2020b). However, it is important to keep in mind that malingering would not necessarily rule out the existence of a psychological disorder (Rogers, 2018). A person who engages in pathological lying could presumably malinger, given the specific context and situation. Therefore, it is important to distinguish features of malingering from pathological lying.

Antisocial Personality Disorder

Deceitfulness is one of the seven diagnostic criteria for ASPD (*DSM-5* 301.7; American Psychiatric Association, 2013). To be diagnosed with ASPD, a minimum of three of seven criteria must be met (American Psychiatric Association, 2013). Thus, deceitfulness is not required to make a diagnosis of ASPD. If deception is present, the *DSM-5* indicates that it is "to gain personal profit or pleasure (e.g., to obtain money, sex, or power)" (American Psychiatric Association, 2013, p. 660). People diagnosed with ASPD are largely males who also have an alcohol use disorder, with the prevalence between 0.2% and 3.3% (American Psychiatric Association, 2013). Our study on pathological liars found a higher prevalence rate, with equal proportion of males and females (Curtis & Hart, 2020b). Further, our assessment study found that most pathological liars did not meet diagnostic criteria for ASPD, often showing remorse and guilt, a lack of aggression, and few having a criminal history or legal problems (Curtis & Hart, 2021a). Last, lies are not required for ASPD, whereas they are the defining and central feature of pathological lying.

Psychopathy

Psychopathy, although not a formal diagnostic entity in the *DSM-5*, has a robust literature documenting its existence. Although some practitioners may view psychopathy as ASPD, Hare (1996) suggested that "most psychopaths . . . meet the criteria for ASPD, but most individuals with ASPD are not psychopaths" (p. 2). Because the key feature of pathological lying is deception, this is true for psychopathy as well (Gillard, 2018). Pathological lying and psychopathy may share the feature of lying, but pathological liars tend to express guilt and remorse for their lies, whereas psychopaths do not (Curtis & Hart, 2020b, 2021c). Further, psychopathy consists of features that are not indicative of pathological lying: lack of remorse, shallow affect, glibness, grandiose self-worth, and failure to accept responsibility. Many pathological liars experience pain and distress from their lies and sometimes seek help from mental health practitioners or forums.

Other Personality Disorders

One of the key distinctions between pathological lying and personality disorders (other than ASPD) is that personality disorders do not have lying as part of the diagnostic criteria. However, this does not preclude people with these personality disorders from lying. For example, people who have narcissistic personality disorder may lie to exaggerate personal features or characteristics (Dike et al., 2005). People with histrionic personality disorder may lie to gain attention (Dike et al., 2005). People with borderline personality disorder may also lie due to patterns of instability (Dike et al., 2005). Dike (2008) claimed that borderline personality disorder is distinct from pathological lying in that falsifications are not usually elaborate and that pathological liars do not show the emotional dysregulation and suicidal behaviors that represent borderline personality disorder.

The presence of lying in conjunction with other problems may be another reason that practitioners provided personality disorder diagnoses to their pathological lying patients (Curtis & Hart, 2021a). Thus, if a person with a personality disorder lies, it is important to assess whether it is the central and pervasive feature of behavior or if it is peripheral to the primary concerns or a function to serve the primary personality issues. Although people with personality disorders may lie, excessive lies are not central to the disorder, as they are to pathological lying.

Substance Use Disorders

Lying and secrets can be found among people who use and abuse substances (Farber et al., 2019; Ford, 1996). People may hide their use from family, friends, coworkers, and law enforcement officers. Lying about a patient's use of drugs or alcohol was in the top six reasons people gave for lying within psychotherapy (Farber et al., 2019). The reason patients lie about substance use is to avoid embarrassment or shame (Farber et al., 2019).

Lying about the use of substances is specific to substance use. In contrast, pathological liars lie about a variety of topics and often tell lies for no reason. In suspected cases of pathological lying, it is important to assess for substance use because confabulations could be the result of a substance-induced persisting amnestic disorder (Dike et al., 2005).

Neurocognitive Disorders

Similar to delusional disorders or psychotic episodes, merely speaking an untruth does not indicate lying. A key feature of neurocognitive disorders is impaired cognitive abilities and functioning (American Psychiatric Association, 2013). An individual who suffers from a neurocognitive disorder may provide information that is not correct or accurate. This does not mean that they are lying because lying requires intent. The misinformation could be due to cognitive decline or impairment in executive functioning.

Brown and colleagues (2017) differentiate lying from confabulation, with specific attention to dementia and neurocognitive disorders. They define confabulation as "the production or creation of false or erroneous memories without the intent to deceive" (p. 1). Thus, false memories are not lying with a deceptive intent. Pathological lying does not consist of organically derived amnesia (Dike et al., 2005). Hence, it is important to rule out neurocognitive disorders when making diagnostic determinations about pathological lying.

Medical Conditions

Dike (2008) discussed other medical conditions that could be confused with pathological lying. He discussed Ganser syndrome as a differential diagnosis of pathological lying. Dike (2008) discussed that elaborate stories or falsehoods are not witnessed in Ganser syndrome, where the seeming lies are confabulations. Ganser syndrome also contains other symptoms that are not found in pathological lying, such as amnesia, hallucinations, sensory changes, and a clouding of consciousness (Dike et al., 2005).

RECOGNITION OF PATHOLOGICAL LYING AS A DIAGNOSTIC ENTITY

The American Psychiatric Association (2021) laid out guidelines for proposals for the addition of a new diagnostic category. The requirements are to provide substantial evidence that the category accomplishes the following:

  (i) Meet criteria for a mental disorder,

  (ii) Have strong evidence of validity,

  (iii) Be capable of being applied reliably,

  (iv) Manifest substantial clinical value (e.g., identify a group of patients now not receiving appropriate clinical attention; facilitate the appropriate use of available treatment[s]),

  (v) Avoid substantial overlap with existing diagnoses, and not be better conceptualized as a subtype of an existing diagnosis, and

  (vi) Have a positive benefit/harm ratio (e.g., acceptable false-positive rate; low risk of harm due to social or forensic considerations). (p. 13)

On the basis of these criteria, we believe that pathological lying warrants being considered a diagnostic entity. Over a century of research and literature in conjunction with our research findings support this notion. In this book and from research findings, we have demonstrated Criteria i through v.

We have indicated within this text and elsewhere that there is a positive benefit to harm ratio (Curtis & Hart, 2021c). People who struggle with pathological lying do not receive a formal diagnosis. The failure to recognize a formal diagnosis complicates treatment and prevents research into further understand pathological lying and exploring effective treatments.

From our research, we know that some individuals who engage in pathological lying will not receive a formal diagnosis and those who do will be granted another diagnosis. Those who receive another diagnosis may either cease psychotherapy or may be provided an ineffective or harmful treatment. There are clearly individuals who are not receiving appropriate clinical attention and their only outlet is through the support of blogs and other media forums. Although support groups have utility and merit, there is certainly a need for mental health practitioners to assist and intervene within cases of pathological lying.

Balancing this perspective, it is certainly important to consider the potential harm from a diagnosis of pathological lying. Psychotherapists do hold negative attitudes toward patients who lie, and this concern could arise in working with pathological lying (Curtis & Hart, 2015, 2021c). We have suggested workshops and education to address this concern (Curtis & Hart, 2021c). We discuss this issue in greater detail in Chapter 9, when considering the therapist's role in working with pathological lying. Another concern could be the stigma attached to the disorder. This concern is largely an issue of whether the patient discusses their diagnosis with others. Further, clinicians can execute their sociopolitical responsibility to educate others about psychopathology, mental health, and specifically about pathological lying (Blashfield & Burgess, 2007). There is evidence that people who struggle with pathological lying are willing to share their problems with others to gain help (Curtis & Hart, 2021b).

Regarding forensic considerations, Dike and colleagues (2005) discussed the case of Judge Couwenberg, who made misrepresentations to become a judge and continued to lie as a judge. A psychiatrist indicated that Judge Couwenberg was suffering from pseudologia fantastica. They stated that

> Judge Couwenberg [was] unfit for judicial service. Although evidence for this latter clarification was not available for review, it is important because for pathological lying to be a desired defense strategy, it must be identified as an illness for which one could be treated and recover fully. Otherwise, the label could be quite damaging to one's reputation and credibility. (p. 347)

They continue to discuss the concerns of psychiatrists offering differing opinions about pathological lying (Dike et al., 2005). Without advancing a diagnostic entity, there is difficulty in forensic assessments and cases. Dike and colleagues (2005) also expressed concerns about no specific psychological tests for pathological lying. In the previous chapter, we provided some assessment data. We also discussed some of our measures that were developed to specifically classify and test for pathological lying (Curtis & Hart, 2020b; Hart, Curtis, & Randell, 2022).

THE RECOGNITION OF A DIAGNOSIS

Dike (2020) stated: "It is long overdue for pathological lying to be accorded the recognition it deserves by mental health clinicians and elevated to a diagnostic entity on its own merits in the *DSM*, complete with a reexamination of its relationship with factitious disorder" (p. 434). We agree with Dike (2008) and many others who came before us. The history and evidence stack up in favor of recognizing pathological lying as a distinct diagnostic entity. Recognition of pathological lying within the *DSM* will be essential for clinicians to make diagnostic determinations, as the *DSM* is one of clinicians' premier tools. Our efforts will be aimed at conducting additional research on pathological lying and to submit it as a diagnostic entity to be recognized within the major nosological systems. Along with the recognition of pathological lying as a diagnostic entity, practitioners could use the definition we have provided, the diagnostic criteria put forth, and the Pathological Lying Inventory (PLI) to help determine a diagnosis. Future research could focus on examining the utility of the diagnostic criteria we recommended and the use of the PLI for making diagnostic decisions. We encourage the investigation of these tools within clinical and forensic practice, as well as developing other useful tools. We continue to explore how this recognition is crucial to helping and treating individuals who exhibit symptoms or pathological lying.

9

Treatment, Clinical Applications, and the Future

S top it! Probably one of the most socially prescribed treatments for any problematic behavior is telling someone to just stop. Think of smoking cigarettes, drinking alcohol, any substance use, overeating, nail-biting, hair-pulling, skin-picking, hoarding, and even anxiety and panic attacks, among others. In many cases involving these behaviors, people, arguably with good intentions, tell individuals to just stop smoking, drinking, or being anxious. The success rates from the social response to just stop usually tends to be low. Lying may often get similar treatment; family or friends may tell someone to just stop lying. We suspect that intervention is not particularly effective.

The entire therapeutic process is aimed at treatment. Assessment and diagnosis are designed to evaluate and determine a person's problem(s). Largely, assessment and diagnosis are aimed at the goal of helping the person resolve, change, modify, or lessen their problem(s). We examine the

https://doi.org/10.1037/0000305-009
Pathological Lying: Theory, Research, and Practice, by D. A. Curtis and C. L. Hart

scant literature and research on treatments for pathological lying. Further, we suggest some potential treatments to be explored within randomized controlled trials (RCTs). Along with treatment, we discuss applications for practitioners and future directions.

FAILURE TO DIAGNOSE COMPLICATES TREATMENT

Proper treatment hinges on a proper diagnosis. Psychotherapeutic interventions are aimed at changing the specific conditions or symptoms for which they were designed. The American Psychological Association (2020a) dictionary defines *treatment* as two things:

1. the administration of appropriate measures (e.g., drugs, surgery, psychotherapy) that are designed to relieve a pathological condition and
2. the intervention to which some participants in an experimental design (the experimental group or treatment group) are exposed, in contrast to a control group, who do not receive the intervention.

If measures are designed to relieve a specific pathological condition and that condition is not recognized, then no treatments would be designed for that condition. Thus, this is one of many reasons to formally recognize pathological lying as a diagnostic entity. A failure to acknowledge pathological lying as a pathological condition or diagnostic entity would logically lead to a failure to develop and offer effective treatments.

The concern of accurately classifying pathological lying and seeking effective treatments is not new. Recall from Chapter 1 that many pioneers in the field recognized the construct of pathological lying, made efforts to study it, and even sought out treatments. Hall (1890) declared that pathological lying cases "demand the most prompt and drastic treatment" (p. 68). Hall suggested that a primary concern for teachers was to recognize pathological lying and apply remedies. However, he further suggested concerns that treatment could be effective in some aspects but potentially aggravate other symptoms. Hall spoke broadly about the prognosis and treatment of pathological liars, but he was more explicit when suggesting "firm responsibility for their acts and words" (p. 70).

As it stands, there has been limited literature and research about the treatment of pathological lying. Dupré (1905) wrote that because the Zeitgeist was not in favor of recognizing pathological lying, interventions would be reserved for the future. He stated:

> But the time is not ripe for such demonstrations, and public opinion still refuses to consider as sick subjects capable of putting such intellectual resources at the service of their perversions. Each age has, relatively speaking, its witchcraft trials; but we can, in the name of the progress already accomplished, foresee in the justice of the future, an intervention more and more broad and more and more fruitful of the forensic psychiatry. (Dupré, 1905, para. 216)

Looking to the future, 100 years later, Dike and colleagues (2005) raised similar concerns and several valid points about the lack of treatment for pathological lying. The failure to recognize pathological lying as a diagnostic entity has influenced the dearth of research. Further, the majority of literature and research on pathological lying is largely that of the late 1800s and early 1900s, some in 1980s, and then a more recent reemerging interest by some scholars. Dike et al. stated:

> The options available for treating pathological lying are also poorly researched. Scientific interest in pathological lying was prominent in the era preceding the development of psychotropic medications, and as a result, the treatment modality discussed consisted mainly of psychotherapy. Even so, the effectiveness of psychotherapy in the treatment of pathological lying has not been systematically studied. (p. 347)

Dike (2008) subsequently emphasized the same concern about pathological lying not being recognized as a diagnostic entity and the consequences of this on research and treatment:

> there are no systematic studies on the effectiveness of psychotherapy in treating PL and no discussion of pharmacotherapy or any other types of interventions. It is possible that there may be a subset of pathological liars for whom pharmacotherapeutic options may help

in reducing impulsivity or the compulsions associated with the urge to lie. In addition, further investigation of CNS [central nervous system] abnormalities may lead to other therapeutic interventions. (para. 17)

Many scholars and practitioners, including us, share these concerns. Other scholars continue to stress the same problem that results from the failure to recognize pathological lying as a diagnostic entity: Ultimately, it hinders research and the delivery of effective treatments. Muzinic et al. (2016) stated:

> To date pathological lying has not been considered as a special diagnosis in classifications, which may be the reason why there are no special guidelines developed to address the foregoing phenomenology. It equally pertains to pharmacotherapy, psychotherapy, or both, indicated for specific symptoms within the foregoing psychiatric entity. (p. 91)

PAST TREATMENTS OF PATHOLOGICAL LYING

While the failure to recognize pathological lying as a diagnostic entity has placed a large stumbling block or wall in the face of research progress into understanding etiology and treatment, some practitioners and scholars have recognized pathological lying as a distinct disorder. In doing so, they have explored outcomes, prognosis, and potential treatments. Within this group of scholars and practitioners, there is a mix of attitudes toward prognosis and treatment, with some being more pessimistic than others about the ability to treat pathological lying.

Anna Stemmermann (1906) presented one of the first dissertations on cases of pathological lying, having evaluated 17 cases in literature and 10 of her own cases (in Healy & Healy, 1915). Stemmermann indicated that the literature did not document much on the prognosis for pathological liars and that such individuals were largely incurable (Healy & Healy, 1915). Stemmermann's work on pathological liars revealed that some patients may do well for a period of years and then revert back to telling excessive lies. With the pessimistic outlook, Stemmermann did argue for a favorable outcome found in one of Delbrück's cases of pathological lying. Stemmermann reported that by applying their *linguistic powers* to being a newspaper editor, the individual was able to have a good prognosis. The idea was one of redirecting the patient's use of language and words toward constructive devices for occupational gain. This notion of treatment can be found in practitioners who may ascribe to ideas of an addictive personality when treating substance abuse. The premise is that people who abuse substances have an addictive personality and will trade one addiction for another. Thus, the therapist may assist the patient in redirecting the addiction toward prosocial behaviors, such as working excessively, an addiction to the gym, or a number of other outlets.

Emil Kraepelin (1912) shared the pessimistic view about the prognosis and treatment of pathological liars: "The prognosis and treatment of the morbid swindler and liar are the same as that indicated in the related forms of the insanity of degeneracy. Many of these patients cause so much trouble that they require permanent custody" (p. 531). It was clear that Kraepelin believed that pathological lying was so problematic, it required some form of isolation, institutionalization, or supervision from others.

Selling (1942) also held a less-than-optimistic perspective on the treatment of pathological lying. Specifically, Selling stated within his definition of pathological lying that "the pathological liar is characterized clinically by a constellation of traits which prevent him from giving full cooperation to the examiner and responding normally to treatment from the point of view of having adequate insight and a normal truth-telling capacity" (p. 336). Thus, Selling appeared to believe that the prognosis would be poor for people who engage in pathological lying because of their lack of motivation and insight, and even inability to be honest.

The pessimistic outlook on change for pathological lying may even extend into the public sector, especially for people who have dealt with pathological lying personally. People who are in relationships with pathological liars struggle with the potential for the individual to make changes. From our study examining blogs and forums of pathological liars (Curtis & Hart, 2021b), one individual who had been in an intimate relationship with a pathological liar for 5 years stated that "they will never be able to tell the truth. Ever! Even with acceptance and therapy, they may continue to lie compulsively. What causes this? I have no idea. Not even doctors know for sure."

Healy and Healy (1915) held a much more optimistic view about prognosis and treatment. They indicated that some of their cases "more or less recovered from a strongly marked and prolonged inclination to falsify," which is imperative to examine for the sake of treatment (p. 7). The Healys presented 24 cases, 12 of which were reported to be cases of pathological lying. From the 12 cases that they reported, Cases 1, 4, and 7 demonstrated "immensely favorable outcome," having a good prognosis or significantly reduced lying in a manner that was no longer causing impairment in functioning or distress (p. 272). The Healys also indicated that several other cases indicated promise. In other cases (e.g., 3, 5, and 6), it appeared that the lying behaviors continued or there was no improvement. With the remaining cases, Healy and Healy did not mention much about treatment or prognosis or stated that it was too early to tell. Let us turn attention to some of these cases to explore past treatments.

In Case 1, Healy and Healy (1915) reported that a 16-year-old girl received a treatment in an institution for delinquent young women. They indicated that over the course of 4 years, she improved. The case broadly claims that her tendencies to lie diminished and attribute some of the success to her mother. The Healys concluded that her lying tendencies were reduced to a minimum and that she had resumed functioning in her life. For Case 4, the authors indicated that 2 years after being removed from her environment, her lying behavior was reduced to occur occasionally; they indicated that she was trustworthy. In Case 7, the general conclusions were that the patient's mother aided in treatment. More specifically, the authors indicated that the onset of pathological lying began shortly after the patient's father caught her masturbating. The masturbatory behaviors followed the patient reportedly taking interest in viewing intimate movie scenes at age 7. The Healys concluded the case by reporting that the patient's resolved sexual habits brought about the resolution of her pathological lying.

Other cases presented by Healy and Healy (1915) consisted of unsuccessful treatments, poor prognosis, or no longitudinal data to assess functioning in later life. For example, Case 2 was stated to reveal no successful treatment and showed delinquent behaviors after being in a corrective institution and Case 3 was discussed as showing an unfavorable prognosis by psychiatrists. Other cases did not mention treatment outcomes explicitly or the case was in the early stages of treatment.

Taken together, Healy and Healy (1915) discussed their concerns of individual differences within each case that affected the prognosis and outcomes. They criticized others who suggested that pathological liars are incapable of being effectively treated or that they were incurable. Instead, Healy and Healy held a more optimistic view of the potential for treatment, citing several cases in which individuals resolved their problematic lying behavior. The Healys also acknowledged the limitations of some of their case studies by discussing how some cases were too recent in research to indicate future or long-term prognoses. They concluded that a total alteration of environmental conditions was necessary for treating pathological lying. They also suggested that family or relatives may be instrumental in the treatment of pathological lying. The authors stressed the importance of physical improvement or physical health as potentially being related to lying behavior. They posited that treatment should include a discussion of "moral failures" in terms of exploring the impact of the patient's lying behaviors on other people (p. 273). They reported that several improved cases were the result of "social foresight" (p. 274). The Healys further stated that directly addressing the lie when it is being told is of great value to treatment of pathological lying.

SUGGESTED TREATMENTS FROM PRACTITIONERS

Several practitioners and scholars have seemed reluctant to stand firm on a specific treatment for pathological lying due to the failure to recognize it as a diagnostic entity. Some authors, more recently, have indicated that some treatments, specifically psychotherapy, may be effective (Gogineni

& Newmark, 2014). Some of the first research to systematically explore a variety of practitioners' suggested treatments for pathological lying can be found in Treanor's (2012) work. She interviewed practitioners and asked them if they have treated someone believed to be a pathological liar then inquired what treatment they use. She reported one example of suggested treatments, which was cognitive behavior therapy (CBT). Treanor stated that while qualitative data were collected about treatment from interviews of practitioners, the summary of the data was beyond the scope of her thesis, and she did not report much on this data. She concluded that long-term psychotherapy was needed and that practitioners should focus on the aftermath of lying rather than preventative measures.

Continuing in this vein, we explored practitioners' suggested treatments for pathological lying. In our study on practitioners' experiences with pathological lying and ability to diagnose, we asked practitioners to suggest a treatment for pathological lying (Curtis & Hart, 2021c). As one might imagine, when asking a diverse group of 295 practitioners about suggested treatment, a variety of treatments were offered (see Figure 9.1; see Appendix D, this volume, for a full list).

Even so, there was a large consensus among practitioners. Most participants (73%) suggested the use of CBT in some form for treatment. About 41% of the clinicians recommended CBT alone as the suggested treatment for pathological lying. Dialectical behavioral therapy, behavioral therapy, acceptance and commitment therapy, emotion-focused therapy, and motivational interviewing were some of the other suggestions that were endorsed by a smaller group of participants. Last, there was a variety of less frequent suggestions that included group psychotherapy, a specific technique (e.g., self-checks and behavioral reminders), or stating that they did not know.

POTENTIAL TREATMENTS

Although the failure to recognize pathological lying as a diagnostic entity has prevented research into exploring the effectiveness of various treatments, there are reasons to consider the use of some treatments and explore their

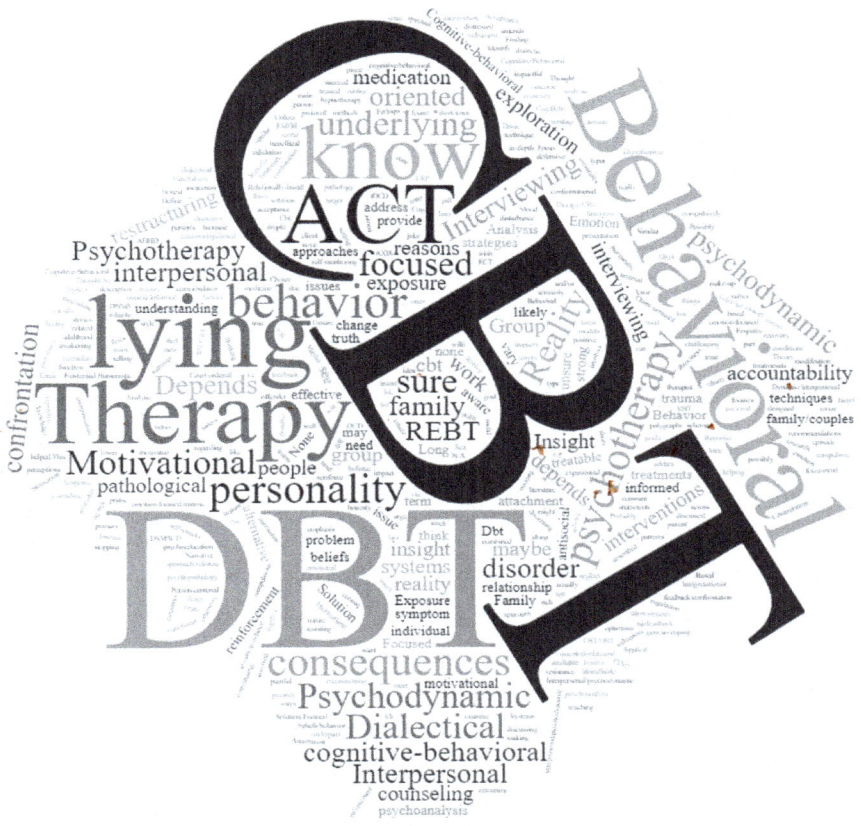

Figure 9.1

Findings from practitioners' suggested treatments. Data from Curtis and Hart (2021c).

effectiveness. As previously discussed, practitioners have largely suggested CBT in some form or fashion for treating pathological lying. We examine the potential applications of CBT for treating pathological lying and review the very limited case studies that have implemented CBT. Along with psychotherapy, specifically CBT, some scant findings of pharmacological treatments are presented. Given the known features and etiology of pathological lying, consideration is given to the theoretical use of other modalities and techniques for treatment.

Cognitive Behavior Therapy

CBT would be a treatment modality worthy of exploration in relation to pathological lying. A robust body of literature supports its use for various psychopathologies (see Beck, 2021). More than 2,000 outcome studies have corroborated CBT's efficacy in treating various psychological disorders and medical issues that have psychological factors (Beck, 2021). The various psychological disorders where CBT has been shown to be effective are published by Division 12 (Society for Clinical Psychology) of the American Psychological Association (2016). Further, CBT has long-term benefits, helping patients prevent or reduce the severity of symptoms or conditions well after psychotherapy (Beck, 2021).

Modell and colleagues (1992) reported the case of a 35-year-old man who identified as a pathological liar. Their study was primarily aimed at brain imaging of pathological lying. Modell and colleagues reported that they did not conduct a posttreatment single-photon emission computerized tomography (SPECT) because the treatment, which was CBT with pharmacotherapy, had no effect on the patient's lying. However, the authors did not provide any specific details about the CBT treatment (e.g., number of sessions, treatment goals). Due to the limited sample ($N = 1$) and lack of details about treatment, it would be careless to conclude CBT is ineffective for treating pathological lying or to foreclose on researching its effectiveness with pathological lying. In fact, other case studies have indicated a favorable response to treatment of pathological lying by use of CBT.

Gogineni and Newmark (2014) discussed CBT in terms of their work with a patient who told stories of building elaborate haunted houses, escaping the police by driving 400 mph over a lake, and an instance of jumping 1 mile from a helicopter into a pool of alligators and sharks to save a friend (p. 451). They reported that the individual had an "underlying negative schema that manifest in the individual's reliance on negative, distorted, and/or rigid and fixated cognitions. These serve to maintain low self-esteem and support the patient's need to seek attention in this manner" (p. 452). Gogineni and Newmark wrote that CBT techniques could be extremely helpful for treating pathological lying. They suggested identifying the situations and cognitions that precede lying behavior in an attempt to identify negative automatic thoughts and distorted thinking. They claimed that resolving negative automatic thoughts tied to low self-esteem could lead to behavioral change. Additional techniques that were reported to be effective were to listen to the lies and stories without a harsh judgment or brash confrontational style and to attend to the patient's underlying mood and affect. In doing so, Gogineni and Newmark reported that the patient's lies decreased and mood improved.

Cognitively, patients could examine beliefs they hold about their self, the world, and the future. As Gogineni and Newmark (2014) suggested, patients could identify and examine the cognitions that occur before their lying behavior. If the lying is viewed as being helpful in the moment for whatever motivation (e.g., to get attention, for a perceived relational gain, to avoid a socially awkward situation, to avoid relational conflict), then these thoughts are worth exploring. As mentioned in previous chapters, people tell lies when they perceive that the truth will not work. If pathological liars hold these perceptions that the truth will not work in many instances, then delving into these thoughts would be critical for the patient and align directly with the CBT model.

If there is a lack of awareness or if the behaviors are reported as impulsive, then therapists could assist the patient in two goals: raising awareness of cognitions that precede a lie or occur while telling a lie, and examining cognitions following the behaviors. It would be useful for patients to explore the cognitions following their lying behaviors, as they have reported feeling pain, remorse, guilt, and shame after telling lies (Curtis & Hart, 2020b). These cognitions would be worth exploring in relation to their lying and how it affects the self and others. Patients who lie pathologically may also have beliefs of helplessness. Our research found that pathological liars state that their lying is out of their control and that they lie for no reason (Curtis & Hart, 2020b). It may be worthwhile to examine these specific beliefs and how they may aid in telling lies.

Another crucial cognition to examine would be how the patient views their own lies. Do they view their lies as bad or immoral? If so, do they experience cognitive dissonance? Or do they deal with dissonance by justifying the lies told? In these cases, the pathological liar may see the outcome as justification for the behavior. In some instances, the hindsight bias may justify the lying behavior. In our study of pathological liars and their writings in blogs (Curtis & Hart, 2021b), we found an example in which telling a lie was justified as a necessary behavior to result in a metamorphosis or some change for the better, which we refer to as a *Phoenix lie*. The anonymous person said

> I have cheated in a past relationship. It was probably the worst thing I've ever done, but I do not regret it. I feel that we both would not be where we are without it. Since then we have communicated about all of the faults of our relationship and have agreed that we were not meant to be with one another. This was my greatest example of lying and deceiving another person.

Developmentally, lies are rarely justified. Children tend to distinguish lie-telling by negatively evaluating antisocial lies and telling prosocial lies with the intention of being polite (Talwar & Lee, 2002a, 2002b; Talwar et al., 2007). Recall that if people lie because they do not think the truth will work, then they are predicting that a lie will be helpful. It is not clear that these predictions are made for pathological liars, and research into this area is warranted. If a person who engages in pathological lying does not consider the consequences of telling the truth or lying, then examining the role of cognitions in regard to moral evaluations of lies may be helpful for patients. For example, are moral evaluations and cognitions about telling a lie considered at the moment a person lies or not until afterward? It is likely that it is the latter, which is why pathological liars feel remorse, guilt, and anxiety after telling lies. Cognitions of moral evaluations occurring following the behavior may lead to guilt. Thus, examining cognitions of morality and the use of types of lies may be useful for a patient.

Behavioral interventions would be equally important. Given that the goal of many pathological liars who want help is to reduce their lying behavior, then behavioral treatments would be worth considering. Learning theory posits that the behavior (lying) would be learned via associations, consequences, and observing the consequences of others (Bandura et al., 1961; Pavlov, 1960; Skinner, 1938). Psychotherapists may conduct a behavioral assessment, exploring antecedents and consequences of the lying behaviors. There is a strong moral prohibition against lying, dating back to early religious and secular texts. Throughout a child's development, lying is often punished and taught to be morally wrong. Parents usually teach their children to be honest, even though the parents themselves lie (Heyman et al., 2009). One study that investigated college students and the lies their parents told found that participants indicated that parents told them to always be honest and truthful, they were punished for lying, and they were never rewarded for lying (Cargill & Curtis, 2017). In some controversial cases, parents have used aversive methods such as using hot sauce or spices on their children's tongues to try to punish their children's lie-telling (Buckholtz, 2004).

Behaviorally, it would be presumed that the pathological liar tells excessive lies because the lies or lie-telling is reinforced more than punished or the reinforcing effects outweigh the punishment. Reinforcement of lies could result from the positive consequences from successfully telling lies (gains, duping delight, attention) or the beneficial outcomes from avoiding being caught telling a lie (avoiding relational conflict or some punishment).

Telling lies can certainly gain the attention of others. Think of the lies told by the patient from Modell and colleagues (1992). The patient discussed constructing a haunted house with dead bodies, jumping out of a helicopter, and going 400 mph to escape the police. It would be difficult for anyone not to attend to lies such as these, even if they knew it was not truthful or were skeptical. It would likely only be some time after hearing numerous lies that a person would shift from attention-giving to disinterest or avoidance of unreliable information. By the time a person has lost interest, the pathological liar could have moved on to gain the attention of others.

One of the core features of the proposed specifier, factitious disorder, is that the attention received from feigning or inducing symptoms is reinforcing. Attention can be a strong reinforcer. Many of the concerns of parents or teachers in working with children's problematic behavior are how the behavior continues or gets worse after disciplining the child. Thus, one potential behavioral solution is omission training, or differential reinforcement of other behaviors (DRO). Omission training or DRO is designed to prevent or rid the appetitive stimulus and result in a decrease in behavior (Domjan, 2003). DRO is preferential to reduce behavior because it does not provide attention to the problematic behavior by delivering an aversive stimulus. Instead, DROs simply ignores the problem behavior and reinforce other desired behaviors. For the child who acts out at school, their acting out is ignored and other behaviors (focusing on a lesson, actively doing schoolwork, staying in the seat, and raising hands) are reinforced by possibly offering stickers, praise, or attention. Reinforcing the desired behaviors will increase their frequency and not attending to the undesired behaviors will reduce their frequency. The use of DRO has been effective within some clinical settings, where decreased behavior was the goal. DRO has been used to decrease toe-walking, trichotillomania, and hand-flapping (Barton et al., 1986; A. Gross et al., 1982; Hirst et al., 2019). Barton and colleagues (1986) used DRO with a child with an intellectual disability to decrease hand-flapping behaviors for a period of 29 days. When the child did not engage in hand-flapping for a 1-minute interval, they would provide reinforcers of juice or sweet fruits. The behavior had been successfully decreased to almost a nonexistent level.

Therefore, DRO could be used with pathological lying. Therapists, family, friends, or even schoolteachers could assist in ignoring the lying behavior and providing reinforcement for other desired behaviors (including being honest). Thom and colleagues (2017) reported successfully using this approach with patients who had pseudologia fantastica; the practitioners showed disinterest in deceptive stories but interest in legitimate ones. Although this may sound easy when discussed, there is a major difficulty with using DRO for lying. Lying, unlike other problematic behaviors (hand-flapping, hair-pulling, skin-picking, acting out in class), is not easily recognized. The clinician would have to accurately distinguish lies from truths, which is a weighty task and one that research indicates is not feasible for most people. Thus, it would be difficult to ignore a lie if you did not know whether the person was lying or being honest. To successfully implement a DRO, one would have to know when the person is lying. Sometimes lies can be revealed through collateral records (Korenis et al., 2015; Newman & Strauss, 2003). Another way to know whether a patient is lying and to show disinterest would be in cases of pseudologia fantastica in which to stories told are impossible or highly improbable (e.g., jumping 1 mile out of a helicopter into a pool of sharks and alligators). In the cases of knowing when the patient is lying, then DRO could be implemented. If solely relying on one's ability to detect deception, then DROs would likely not be the best option because people are not effective lie detectors. In these cases, a potentially better, more pragmatic route for a patient may be to examine the antecedents and consequences of their lies and related cognitions.

The outcome studies on the efficacy and effectiveness of CBT as a treatment for pathological lying are scant, and much work is needed in this area. The robust empirical support for CBT with treating other psychological disorders along with it being the primary treatment suggested by practitioners to treat pathological lying warrants continued investigation. Researchers and practitioners are strongly encouraged to conduct RCTs with CBT for pathological lying.

Habit Reversal Training

If the patient indicates lying behavior is so impulsive that it tends to be done without much cognitive awareness, then another behavioral package to consider would be that of habit reversal training (HRT). HRT is a behavioral therapy technique that consists of raising awareness about the behavior and the urges to engage in the behavior, offering a competing response, and relaxation training. HRT has been successful in treating a variety of impulse and repetitive behavioral disorders, such as trichotillomania, Tourette syndrome, tics, stuttering, and nail-biting (Bate et al., 2011; Farhat et al., 2020; Himle et al., 2006).

Our research has indicated that pathological liars tend to report telling lies for no reason and that there is a compulsive aspect to telling lies (Curtis & Hart, 2020b). Other literature we have reviewed has also indicated that pathological lying may be impulsive (e.g., Modell et al., 1992). If a patient with pathological lying reports lies being told impulsively, then there may be a need to raise awareness for the patient pertaining to when and where they tell lies and have urges to lie. Then, the therapist and patient could work together to identify competing responses that could be executed instead of the lying behaviors. Pathological liars also indicate that lies reduce anxiety in the situation (Curtis & Hart, 2020b), thus relaxation training could be explored as a means to help patients deal with their anxiety in social situations when telling the truth may seem problematic.

Couples, Family, or Group Therapy

As pathological lying is largely a behavior that occurs in relational contexts and typically impairs social functioning, then it would be remiss to not consider treatment modalities that are largely relational: couples, family, or group psychotherapy. Ford (1996) stated that "because lying is a social phenomenon, the spouse or other family members may also need to be involved in the treatment plan" (p. 238). We agree with this contention. It may be that a patient who is family or relationally mandated for treatment by an ultimatum may need to consider, at minimum, bringing in another person in service of that patient's treatment plan. Also, the patient may want to consider couples, family, or group psychotherapy in conjunction with individual psychotherapy. Garlipp (2017) suggested "augmenting individual therapy with couple or family therapy session should be considered" (p. 326). Others have stated that it is imperative for the treatment of pathological liars to have stable relationships and social support (Korenis et al., 2015).

Dimitrakopoulos and colleagues (2014) reported on a case of pseudologia fantastica and folie à deux. They reported a favorable outcome for the patient at a 1-year follow-up, which was attributed to a community mental health setting that provided individual psychotherapy and a family approach. The authors stated that the context helped the patient by decreasing the telling fantasy stories and admitting to telling excessive lies.

Couples and family psychotherapy would be useful to consider when an individual's lies have taken a toll on those relationships. The systems approach could be a means for the patient to examine, firsthand, the consequences their lies have for others they love and care about. Additionally, the couple could work together to identify the interaction cycle and find ways to cease or change interactions that may encourage or foster lying from the individual who lies excessively.

All these therapeutic modalities could also be beneficial from increasing the patient's awareness about lying without the confrontation of the therapist. Group is specifically useful for providing a space for others to be confrontational (Yalom & Leszcz, 2020). Confrontation from others could preserve the therapeutic relationship and allow the therapist to comment on the process and explore the function and consequences of the lies. If a pathological liar were in a general process group, then consensual validation of how the lying behavior appeared to affect others may prove useful. A homogenous group with pathological lying as its theme could also provide some utility for universalism and support, which may allow members to discuss their lying behaviors without concern of shame or guilt (Yalom & Leszcz, 2020).

Like all treatment modalities for pathological lying, it is an area that has limited research and needs further investigation. Although the one study previously mentioned (Dimitrakopoulos et al., 2014) pertained to pseudologia fantastica and folie à deux, it indicated promise with individual and family therapy. Given that lying often impairs social functioning and lies require communication with others, these modalities are worth further consideration.

Potential Pharmacological Treatments

As with psychotherapy, there has been limited research on the effectiveness of pharmacological treatments for pathological lying. As Dike and colleagues (2005) stated, "Scientific interest in pathological lying was prominent in the era preceding the development of psychotropic medications, and as a result, the treatment modality discussed consisted mainly of psychotherapy" (p. 347). Dike et al. suggested, in reference to B. H. King and Ford's (1988) findings related to pathological lying and central nervous system abnormalities, that there may be a role for pharmacotherapy. They suggested that future research should explore pharmacotherapy and psychotherapy in combination for the treatment of pathological lying. In a more pointed direction, Dike (2008) suggested research on pharmacotherapy for impulsivity or compulsive behaviors.

In addition to B. H. King and Ford's (1988) findings, other neuroscience research has implicated the thalamus, decreased gray–white matter ratios, and increased white matter in the orbitofrontal cortex (Modell et al., 1992; Yang et al., 2005, 2007). Modell and colleagues (1992) reported that the individual case they observed had undergone treatment of fluoxetine (120 mg/d), lithium (0.6–0.8 mEq/L), and CBT, although they indicated that the treatment had no effect on the patient's lying.

Gogineni and Newmark (2014) believed that pharmacological interventions were largely ineffective. They stated that "psychopharmacology has limited value in treatment of pseudologia fantastica symptoms" (p. 454). They reported that the patient was prescribed methylphenidate, amphetamine salts, quetiapine, risperidone, and selective serotonin reuptake inhibitors but was currently taking lisdexamfetamine, paliperidone, s-citalopram, oxcarbazepine, and testosterone gel. It is important to note that the patient had several diagnoses (posttraumatic stress disorder, oppositional defiant disorder, attention-deficit/hyperactivity disorder— combined type, child sexual abuse, and Klinefelter syndrome). Thus, the various medications were likely aimed at treating a variety of symptoms and concerns. However, Gogineni and Newmark (2014) did not specifically indicate how they concluded that psychopharmacology was limited with the patient.

Although Modell and colleagues (1992) reported that combined treatments of pharmacotherapy and psychotherapy did not yield any benefits, there are many more questions that suggest this area may be ripe for further research. Thus, given the dearth of research in this area and the literature largely occurring before the development and refinement of many psychotropic medications, we encourage continued research into the area of psychopharmacological treatments for pathological lying.

CLINICAL APPLICATIONS

One of the most important clinical applications is to accurately understand that most people do not lie often (Serota et al., 2010; Serota & Levine, 2015). Further, most patients do not lie often (Curtis & Hart, 2020a).

Reading literature on deception could very well make deception salient. A mistake of peril would be lie bias—that is, to err by assuming that most patients lie often. The pendulum could easily swing the other direction, for practitioners and academics, when the assumption is that everyone lies. Some authors claim that deception in psychotherapy is frequent, pervasive, and commonplace (e.g., Ford, 1996). In fact, it is from the findings that most people are honest that the theoretical framework for investigating pathological lying was inspired.

In the case of a pathological liar, they do lie frequently. However, the majority of patients are not pathological liars. Additionally, the lying frequency of pathological liars within a psychotherapeutic context, when seeking help, has not yet been examined. In an assessment study we conducted, the participants were asked at the end of the clinical interview "What did you lie about in our meeting today?" (Curtis & Hart, 2021a). The participants collectively reported that they did not lie to the interviewer. One reason given for not lying to the interviewer was that "I know my lying is toxic and I'm trying to help [the researchers learn more about pathological lying]"; another participant indicating having "no reason," and another participant indicated trying to be truthful by "forcing myself" because it is a "scientific study." With that, one participant did report lying to the interviewer about the participant's sister being athletic. Thus, a practitioner may need to consider one's position, attitudes, and whether the patient is a pathological liar.

Psychotherapists generally hold a truth bias (Curtis, 2013; Kottler & Carlson, 2011). Why would anyone spend money, dedicate their precious time, and exert effort to enter psychotherapy only to lie? This bias is largely positioned in the right direction, in that most patients are not lying most of the time. However, it is a myth that clients are always honest, and this is often perpetuated by psychotherapists and supervisors (Kottler & Carlson, 2011). Further, practitioners are rarely trained in deception within psychotherapy, and training programs do not often give this area attention (Curtis, 2013). The lack of communication about dishonesty within psychotherapy likely advances the patient honesty myth and strengthens the truth bias. Although the truth bias largely matches reality, the risks of assuming all patients are honest is naivety, the consequences of being duped, and positioning oneself to avoid helping a pathological liar work through their lies.

Although most patients are honest most of the time, it certainly does not discount the feeling of being duped by a patient or dealing with a patient who is a pathological liar. It is important for clinicians to consider the role of the practitioner and biases held. If lying becomes salient and noticed often (or even sought after), then truth bias may transition into a lie bias. A truth bias swinging toward a lie bias may provide some utility for seeking out lies but still poses problems, specifically for the therapeutic alliance. Additionally, assuming that most people are lying most of time would surely lead to false-positive errors. Thus, we suggest caution when exploring lying in therapy. If one does find that they have been duped, they should resist the conclusion that lying occurs more frequently than it does. Additionally, we encourage clinicians to accept lying as a part of therapy (Kottler & Carlson, 2011).

Therapeutic Alliance

Clinicians are usually drawn to the profession because they want to be helpers. Helping within psychotherapy largely hinges on the relationship—specifically, the therapeutic alliance. It has been suggested that the key component of helping someone who is a pathological liar is to establish rapport and develop a robust therapeutic alliance (Ford, 1996).

There is a critical balance between believing one's client and being allowed to explore, examine, and challenge. Empathy and truth bias can diminish the therapist's ability to discover whether the patient is being dishonest (Newman & Strauss, 2003; Pankratz, 1998). This position can lead one to being duped and the consequences that come with it. Deception has the potential to destroy trust and undermine the therapeutic relationship. Our work has found that psychotherapists hold numerous negative attitudes upon discovering patient's lies (Curtis & Hart, 2015). People do not generally like being on the receiving end of deception. For the psychotherapist, it is important to distance oneself from viewing the lie as a personal attack and instead examine the function of the lie. Let your compassion override your defensiveness. While being compassionate, keep your wits, skepticism, and inquisitive stance.

The role of the psychotherapist is not the same as that of an interrogator or detective. Newman and Strauss (2003) noted that "unlike police detectives who interrogate suspects, or trial attorneys who cross-examine witnesses, therapists generally search for relevant information in a more collaborative fashion with their clients" (p. 243). Relatedly, Kottler and Carlson (2011) stated that "it really isn't our job to play detective or interrogator and determine what is true" (p. 278). The approach of interrogators or detectives could be potentially damaging to the therapeutic relationship. Regarding lies within psychotherapy, Barnett (2011) cautioned therapists that "taking the attitude or approach of an interrogator and believing nothing until I receive absolute proof would likely be inimical to the establishment and maintenance of a positive therapeutic alliance" (p. 125).

Although therapists are not interrogators or detectives, they share some commonalities. Psychotherapists receive pieces of the puzzle and attempt to put it together cohesively. Further, the core of what psychotherapists do is ask questions, which can feel like an interrogation. The imagery of a detective or interrogator tends to be connected to seeking out information in a small room, often without regard for the person. Additionally, the information a detective or interrogator seeks is usually tied to legal consequences for the person. Thus, when it is said that therapists are not interrogators or detectives, what is meant is that the relationship is not merely a means to gain information to determine the ground truth. For psychotherapy, the relationship is the key by which information is learned in an attempt to help the individual. Thus, by working toward a positive therapeutic alliance, the patient may confess the lies told more openly and be better equipped to examine the function of those lies.

Addressing the Lie

So, if one is not an interrogator, then how should a practitioner handle lies within psychotherapy? Should you confront the lie or let it go? Can you raise awareness about the problem (excessive lying) if you never address the behavior or fail to recognize it (lies) within the therapeutic context? Thom and colleagues (2017) suggested two possible avenues for dealing with pathological lying in treatment: to confront the person when they lie or to show disinterest in the lie while keeping interest in the patient. However, Thom and colleagues claimed that clinicians, in response to discovering that they have been lied to, would likely confront the lie in a harsh or punitive manner, which may turn the patient away. Ford (1996) cautioned the same and stated that establishing rapport "does not necessarily mean a frontal attack on the lying behavior" (p. 238). Instead, Ford (1996) suggested that a nonconfrontational approach would be more effective.

From a behavioral perspective, confronting the lie could potentially be reinforcing or punishing, depending on how it is done. Think back to the interrogator who only wants information from the person for some other means and not for the benefit of the individual. A harsh, shameful, or belittling confrontation could be punishing. However, an unintended consequence could be that the patient would want to avoid future punishment from revealing lying behaviors, resulting in seeking out another therapist. Another potential concern of a confrontation would be that it provides attention to the lie-telling behavior, potentially reinforcing it.

One approach would be to provide positive feedback or reinforcement to the patient for the courage to discuss the lie (Farber et al., 2019). Thus, the clinician would not be reinforcing the lie but the patient's willingness to honestly discuss and examine the lie. This route would likely avoid a shameful response to confronting a lie and encourage more open dialogue and investigation about the function of lies.

Along these lines, another alternative to a confrontation of the lie would be for the therapist to raise awareness of the lying behavior. Encouraging disclosure could increase awareness and would allow the therapist and patient to explore the function of the lies from a more detached stance of understanding the behavior and cognitions rather than a punitive or shaming position. If the goal was to raise awareness, then HRT should be considered. For HRT, the patient is responsible for recognizing their lying behavior. Within HRT, the markers to raise awareness about the behavior are neutral, to reduce positive or negative associations. It is imperative not to shame a person further for telling lies when raising awareness about lying behavior. Similarly, it is important not to foster a positive association for the patient with the behavior that is desired to be reduced (i.e., lying).

Hollender and Hersh (1970) suggested another alternative. They indicated that the therapist cannot serve the role of detective and helper. They stated that assuming dual roles often results in a failure. They claimed that the roles should be separated, with the primary care physician confronting the patient and their lies (interrogator/detective) so that the therapist does not have to confront the patient and can remain in the helper role (Hollender & Hersh, 1970).

Other than addressing the lie, Thom et al. (2017) also suggested not giving attention to the lie while maintaining interest in the patient. Does this approach sound like anything we have already mentioned? This would be akin to implementing DRO. This could very well be executed if the lies were known. Drawing from what was previously discussed, the therapist could praise the courage to discuss lies while not showing any interest in the content of the stories or lies themselves.

Overall, an abrupt confrontation is not likely to be as effective as raising awareness and exploring the function of the lie and the cognitions related to the lie. Thus, the therapist's role is to follow patients' lead because they are in charge of what is shared or hidden (Kottler & Carlson, 2011). Having discussions about psychotherapy within the informed consent and the process of discovery for the sake of the patient may assist the patient with discussing lies. One of the take-home points from Farber et al. (2019) for dealing with deception in psychotherapy is to encourage clinicians to discuss the process of disclosure before asking a patient to disclose. Discussing the expectation and value of the disclosure process will equip patients to anticipate negative affect or a desire to avoid examining the lie (Farber et al., 2019). If the patient is engaged in CBT and expects to examine the antecedents and consequences of behavior while examining the beliefs and thoughts related to lying, then it would be expected that a therapist would take time to examine a lie with the patient. All of the foundational work of discussing the process of disclosure and what to expect with psychotherapy will be paramount for examining the lies within psychotherapy.

A confrontation could lead to resistance, whereas a mutual exploration would be a collaborative effort to examine the behavior and decide whether change should be made. Therefore, discussing one's role and the nature of psychotherapy upfront is not only an ethical practice but also allows the patient to anticipate discussing lies from a position of growth rather than a punitive position.

Quid Pro Quo

Given that we expect honesty (or complete honesty) from patients, are we expected to deliver such honesty in return? Or do therapists hold a position of hypocrisy, expecting patients to be completely forthcoming yet not reciprocating with honesty? The hypocrisy around lying has been evidenced in other relationships. In intimate relationships, people expect their romantic partners to be honest while finding it acceptable to tell lies themselves (Hart et al., 2014). Within parental relationships, the same hypocrisy is found, where parents encourage their children to be completely honest and then do not practice what is being taught (Heyman et al., 2009; Williams et al., 2013). Deception can be found within other health care relationships, such as physicians and nurses lying to patients (Fallowfield et al., 2002; Haw & Stubbs, 2010; Jackson, 2001; Olsen, 2012; Palmieri & Stern, 2009; Tavaglione & Hurst, 2012; Teasdale & Kent, 1995).

The reality is that therapists are not always honest with their patients. Therapists tell their patients lies, mostly with a beneficent intent (Curtis & Hart, 2015). In addition to lying with the desire to help the patient, psychotherapists may lie due to their own frustrations or because they like or dislike the patient (Farber et al., 2019). Even though deception in psychotherapy occurs, it is perceived by the general public and by psychotherapists to largely be unethical behavior (Curtis & Kelley, 2020b). Thus, within psychotherapy there appears to be the same relational pattern of the expectation for honesty in one direction, patient to therapist.

Knowing that clinicians are not immune from lying behavior could remind the clinician to examine the function of the lie rather than taking a purely defensive stance toward being lied to. Additionally, the practitioner could consider self-disclosure of their own lying behavior in an attempt to model the examination of lies within psychotherapy. This recommendation would have the caveat of considering the lie, the therapeutic alliance, and that it is intended only to model the process rather than become a therapeutic intervention for the therapist.

FUTURE DIRECTIONS

The obvious direction for the future is to recognize pathological lying as a diagnostic entity within major nosological systems. The process is currently halted at diagnosis. A formal recognition of pathological lying removes the clinical and research roadblock that has been in place for more than a century. Clinically, the failure to formally recognize pathological lying as a diagnostic entity leads to the absence of treatment or using treatment interventions that may be ineffective or even harmful. A formal recognition of pathological lying would promote more research into exploring its etiology and effective treatments. As it stands, many people are struggling with their lying behaviors, and it is taking a toll on them and their relationships. To this end, clinicians are unable to recognize their difficulties as they are and cannot suggest treatments that are backed by research. It is clear that the recognition of pathological lying would promote much more benefit to individuals who have been and continue to struggle.

There is a dire need to recognize what psychiatrists, psychologists, and mental health professionals have long known. Pathological lying is not a behavior that only occurred more than a century ago. More and more individuals are finding platforms to discuss their difficulties with lying. From one blog, Tugaleva (2013) insightfully stated:

> The more I've told my story and the more I've helped others tell their stories, the more I've realized that the girl I used to be isn't just an embarrassing memory to sweep under the carpet. My lies were fueled by a desperate hunger for love and acceptance—a hunger that runs silently and rampantly through our society, destroying our courage

and our relationships with one another. If we're ever going to be happy, we must come back to the truth about ourselves. That journey starts individually. It starts with accepting and sharing those facets of the human condition that we all know about but are too afraid to share. The parts of our past that make us cringe are, paradoxically, the very parts of ourselves that we should be showing to people. . . . We love to see others displaying the courage it takes to be true, honest, and authentic because it gives us all that same courage. If you're struggling for authenticity, struggling to live a completely honest existence, I'll share with you a secret: it gets easier. It gets easier not just because of practice but also because you'll inspire people with your willingness to go out there and be yourself in a world that is constantly bombarding you with ready-made formulas for how to be someone else. And if there's one thing I've learned from my experiences as both a pathological liar and an authentic human being, it's this: inspiring people is much more worthwhile than shocking them.

Where can people go to discuss their behaviors, difficult emotions, and thoughts if not to a mental health practitioner? Recognition of pathological lying provides those who suffer a venue to discuss, learn, and examine the behavior with mental health professionals.

Along with recognition of pathological lying as a diagnostic entity, we encourage a proliferation of research in the area. Throughout this book, we have laid out several areas that are worth investigation. One theoretical model worth examining is that of the biopsychosocial model of psychopathology. The biopsychosocial model has been adopted by the fifth edition of the *Diagnostic and Statistical Manual of Mental Disorders* and can be used by various practitioners and researchers (American Psychiatric Association, 2013).

The evidence laid out in this book highlights findings of pathological lying at each level of analysis of the bio (e.g., biological findings of white–gray matter and central nervous system abnormalities), psycho (e.g., thoughts, behaviors, emotions), and social (e.g., relationships) model. At the biological level, there is certainly a dearth of neuroscience research related to pathological lying. At the psychological level of analysis, cognitions, behaviors, emotions, and development can be further investigated.

For example, are there common core beliefs found among pathological liars? Are there consistent behavioral antecedents or consequences that shape the lying behavior? Are lies reinforced more than punished for pathological liars, or is there a lack of insight into consequences? Is the lie-telling behavior reinforced through attention? Is lying reinforced by reducing in-the-moment anxiety or negative affect? Does emotion regulation influence telling lies?

Developmentally, what cognitions and behaviors are present within the years of childhood or adolescence when lying and theory of mind are evidenced? What is the developmental trajectory that influences normative lie-telling versus pathological lying? Talwar and Crossman (2011) discussed theory of mind as it may relate to the developmental trajectories of prosocial and antisocial lies, where cognitive sophistication is required to imagine how others may feel. They also suggested that the developmental trajectory of normative lying may follow an inverted U-shape, where lying increases in elementary education when cognitive abilities are developing and subsequently decrease due to the socialization process of lying being a generally unfavorable behavior. Lavoie, Yachison, et al. (2017) found evidence that age and theory of mind was able to differentiate various lying behaviors (e.g., being honest, polite lies, instrumental lies, dual lies). Those with a low theory of mind and who were younger tended to be instrumental liars. The researchers suggested that instrumental liars may represent an earlier phase within the lie-telling developmental trajectory. Continuing to explore developmental trajectories of lie-telling behavior, Lavoie, Leduc, et al. (2017) examined 229 children, aged 3 to 14 years, and found three classes of liars: occasional (51%), instrumental (42%), and antisocial (7%). The antisocial liars represented the highest frequency of lies for avoiding punishment, blaming others, and protecting the self. Additionally, older children with low theory of mind were more likely to be classified as antisocial liars. These findings indicate a developmental trajectory of lying behavior, where most children, as they develop, tell fewer lies. However, some older children that have a delayed development of theory of mind may still engage in telling numerous lies. Are some of these children pathological liars? Examining developmental trajectories and cognitive, behavioral, and social factors may enhance our understanding of the development of pathological lying and provide a basis for treatment and intervention.

There are other various areas worthy of investigation. For example, researchers may explore the use of other psychological tests or measures (e.g., Structured Interview of Reported Symptoms—2nd Edition; Personality Assessment Inventory) with a pathological lying sample. Additional facets of specifiers might also be examined. For example, do pathological liars with a pseudologia fantastica specifier tell lies with a greater magnitude than those who do not tell fantastic stories? Clinically, RCTs are needed to examine the effectiveness of psychological and pharmacotherapy treatments.

CONCLUSION

Pathological liars are not dark, exploitative, calculating monsters who seek every opportunity to hoodwink and exploit others for their own selfish gains. They tend to be individuals who struggle with communicating honestly. They recognize that their behaviors cost them relationships and lead them to feel guilt or shame. Many want and seek out help. Historically, the harm to pathological liars (and their loved ones) has manifested in two ways: failure to recognize their behavior as pathological and stereotypically painting the picture of pathological liars as lacking remorse for their actions. One begets the other. By recognizing pathological lying as a distinct disorder, it can be further understood, and the negative societal stereotype can be amended. As research has further explored pathological lying, we have learned that these individuals do show remorse, feel guilt and shame, and are anxious after telling lies.

Many people who engage in pathological lying (and those with whom they are in relationship) want help. They want to understand the reasons for their behavior and prevent it from ruining relationships. The failure to recognize pathological lying as a diagnostic entity is not just a failure for nosology; it is a failure to help people and their loved ones who are suffering. The pains from pathological lying are not just felt with the individual but usually outpour into their relationships, their families, and society at large.

To close on a message of hope: We hope that our research efforts and attempts to synthesize the scattered writings of pathological lying will renew interest in this area. Specifically, we hope to inspire researchers to pick up the gauntlet and conduct studies on the etiology, accurate assessment, and effective treatments of pathological lying. Our work will equip researchers to initiate systematic studies on the effectiveness of psychotherapy in treating pathological lying. Researchers may explore how clinicians could best work with pathological liars within clinical settings. Research could also examine the forensic implications and applications for pathological lying. We hope to pick up the torch carried by the prolific scholars and giants who came before us. These great authors recognized the concerns of pathological lying and deemed it an area worthy of dedicating time, writing, practice, and research. We hope our work will provide insight for practitioners, researchers, and those who engage in pathological lying. We believe we have provided tools, definitions, and assessments for researchers to further investigate numerous avenues in understanding and better helping pathological liars. Ultimately, we hope to better understand and more effectively help those who suffer with pathological lying.

Appendix A:
Survey of Pathological Lying (SPL)
From Curtis and Hart (2020b)[1]

1 (*strongly disagree*) to 7 (*strongly agree*) for Items 1–7

1. My lying behaviors have resulted in impairment for me in
    a. my occupation.
    b. social relationships.
    c. finances.
    d. legal contexts.
2. My lying causes me significant distress.
3. My lying has put myself or others in danger.
4. My lying is something out of my control.
5. After I lie, I feel less anxious.
6. My lies tend to grow larger from an initial lie.
7. Most of the lies I tell are for no reason.

---

[1]Reprinted from "Pathological Lying: Theoretical and Empirical Support for a Diagnostic Entity," by D. A. Curtis and C. L. Hart, 2020, *Psychiatric Research and Clinical Practice*, 2(2), supplementary material (https://doi.org/10.1176/appi.prcp.20190046). CC BY 4.0.

8. What is the earliest stage that you or others considered yourself to be a pathological liar?

Childhood (3–10 years)

Adolescence (10–20 years)

Early adulthood (20–40 years)

Middle adulthood (40–60 years)

Late adulthood (65 years or more)

9. How long have you been telling numerous lies or engaged in pathological lying?

3 months

6 months

1 year

1–5 years

More than 5 years

Appendix B:
Pathological Lying Inventory From Hart, Curtis, and Randell (2022)[1]

33 Items

1–7 Likert: 1 = *strongly disagree* to 7 = *strongly agree*

Excessive/pervasive ($\alpha = .906$)

1. I lie much more than most people.
2. I lie a lot.
3. If people knew how much I lied, they would be surprised.
4. My lying occurs across various contexts.
5. I have a consistent habit of lying.
6. Despite the situation, I often find myself lying.
7. I lie too much.
8. I am surprised at how often I lie.

---

[1]From *Pathological Lying Inventory*, by C. L. Hart, D. A. Curtis, and J. A. Randell, 2022, Christian L. Hart, Ph.D. (https://christianlhart.com/pli). Copyright 2022 by Human Deception Laboratory. Reprinted with permission.

Compulsion/pointless nature ($\alpha = .843$)

1. Often, I have no idea why I am lying.
2. My lies sometimes seem to have no point.
3. When I lie, there is often no clear motive.

Functioning ($\alpha = .912$)

1. My lying causes problems in my social relationships.
2. My lying causes problems in my romantic life.
3. My lying causes problems in my friendships.
4. My lying causes problems with my family.
5. My lying causes problems in my work or school life.
6. My lying disrupts my life.

Distress ($\alpha = .923$)

1. Life would be much better if I didn't lie so much.
2. My lying makes me miserable.
3. My lying causes me distress.
4. I would be much happier if I could stop lying.
5. My lying causes me a great deal of sadness.
6. My lying makes me feel crazy.
7. My lying causes me pain.
8. I can't stand my lying.

Risk ($\alpha = .873$)

1. Lying causes many bad things to happen to me.
2. My lying causes me to harm others or to put them at risk.
3. My lying sometimes puts me in danger.
4. My lying causes me to lose opportunities.
5. My lying has caused me to lose freedoms.

Persistent ($\alpha = .911$)

1. My lying has been an issue for a long time.
2. I've noticed my habit of lying for over six months.
3. For most of my adult life, I've noticed my habit of lying.

Appendix C:
Therapists' Diagnosis

If you provided a diagnosis, what diagnosis?

Responses	Frequency
Clarification—I do not make clinical diagnosis. The individual did [to] qualify for special ed.	1
ADHD	1
ADHD and oppositional defiant disorder	1
ADHD; personality disorder NOS	1
Anorexia nervosa	1
Antisocial PD	1
Antisocial and or borderline PD	1
Antisocial PD	1
Antisocial PD, narcissistic PD	1
Antisocial personality	1
Antisocial PD	7
Antisocial PD or conduct disorder	1
Anxiety, depression, high expressed emotion in family	1
Antisocial PD	2

(continues)

Responses	Frequency
Autism spectrum disorder and borderline PD	1
Attachment disorder, borderline PD	1
ADHD	1
Autism based on IDEA criteria	1
Bipolar disorder	1
Bipolar disorder	3
Bipolar disorder	2
Bipolar disorder II	1
Bipolar disorder I	1
Borderline	2
Borderline or antisocial PD	1
Borderline PD	1
Borderline PD	4
Borderline PD	3
Borderline PD, R/O bipolar disorder	1
Borderline PD	1
Borderline personality traits	1
Borderline PD	1
Cannot remember	1
Cluster B PD	1
Cluster B PD	1
Conduct disorder	1
Depends on person; most commonly PD but often complex PTSD or dissociation	1
Depends on the case	1
Depression	1
Depressive diagnosis	1
Eating disorder and depression	1
Emotional disturbance	1
Emotional disturbance	2
Emotional disturbance	1
Alcohol use disorder, severe	1
F32.9 (major depressive disorder, single episode)	1
F419 (anxiety disorder)	1
Generalized anxiety disorder, major depressive disorder	1

(*continues*)

Responses	Frequency
Impulse control disorder	2
Major depression, alcohol abuse, possible ADD	1
Major depressive disorder	1
Major depressive disorder, borderline PD	1
Mixed PD	1
n/a	1
n/a	1
Narcissistic	1
Narcissistic or antisocial PD, R/O delusional disorder	1
Narcissistic PD	3
Narcissistic PD	3
Narcissistic, borderline, dependent, antisocial, other Axis II diagnoses (*DSM-IV*)	1
Obsessive compulsive disorder	1
Obsessive compulsive PD	1
Obsessive compulsive disorder, unspecified	1
Oppositional defiant disorder, antisocial PD	1
Opiate use disorder	1
Oppositional defiant disorder	1
PD	1
PD	3
PD	1
PD	1
PD NOS Cluster B and C features, anxiety-based disorders	1
PD, NOS	1
PD	1
Psychopathy	1
PTSD	1
PTSD	1
Qualified for an emotional disturbance in school setting—outside diagnosis from different clinician	1
Schizophrenia based on past history of criminal records	1
Sociopath, narcissistic	1
Some, not all; antisocial PD	1
Stimulant use disorder, malingering	1

(continues)

Responses	Frequency
Substance abuse	1
Substance abuse, gambling addiction, PD	1
Substance use disorder	1
This case was one or two couples sessions where lying was the presenting issue	1
Usually pedophiles or sex addicts or addicts of any type	1
Usually PDs because pathological lying is not in the *DSM*	1
Usually PTSD, depressive disorder NOS, antisocial traits, borderline or narcissistic PD	1
Varied, narcissistic PD, borderline PD, schizophrenia, bipolar disorder	1
Varied, substance abuse, PDs	1
Total	75

Note. ADD = attention-deficit disorder; ADHD = attention-deficit/hyperactivity disorder; *DSM* = *Diagnostic and Statistical Manual of Mental Disorders*; IDEA = Individuals With Disabilities Education Act; n/a = not available; NOS = not otherwise specified; PD = personality disorder; PTSD = posttraumatic stress disorder; R/O = rule out.

Appendix D:
Therapists' Suggested Treatments

What treatment(s) do you believe may be effective for someone who suffered from pathological lying?

Responses	Frequency
?	1
A range of psychotherapy approaches could be beneficial	1
Acceptance and commitment therapy	1
Accountability; not aware of reliable "treatment protocol" available	1
ACT	2
ACT, CBT, psychodynamic	1
ACT, DBT	2
Address underlying fears of the truth	1
Analysis of each episode	1
Applied behavior analysis through problem-solving and teaching Alternative ways to obtain outcome	1
Behavioral	2
Behavioral	1
Behavioral—practice as in exposure therapy	1

(continues)

Responses	Frequency
Behavioral: reinforce honesty	1
Behavioral modification	1
Behavioral or systems therapy	1
Behavioral, systems	1
Behavioral, with strong, impactful, maybe painful consequences for lying; then CBT	1
Biofeedback, CBT, journaling, making amends to people	1
CBT	1
CBT	1
CBT	25
CBT and solution focused	1
CBT and interpersonal	1
CBT, DBT, ACT	1
CBT or DBT	1
CBT, attachment, behavioral, solution focused, DBT	1
CBT and DBT	1
CBT and DBT, and family systems	1
CBT and DBT for emotion regulation	1
CBT, DBT, and holistic approaches	1
CBT, DBT, interpersonal	1
CBT, DBT, psychodynamic, and client-centered	1
CBT, existential/humanistic, exposure to consequences?	1
CBT, medication?	1
CBT, psychoanalysis, family/couples	1
CBT, RBT, short-term trauma focused, solution focused	1
CBT, REBT, ACT	1
CBT, systems, MI	1
CBT; family therapy; marriage counseling	1
CBT, interpersonal, analytic	1
CBT, DBT, solution focused	1
CBT, alternative medicine	1
CBT, group psychotherapy	1
Cognitive-behavioral interventions	1
Cognitive	1

(*continues*)

Responses	Frequency
Cognitive	1
Cognitive and cognitive behavioral	1
CBT	1
Cognitive behavioral	4
Cognitive behavioral	5
Cognitive behavioral	4
Cognitive behavioral and DBT	1
Cognitive behavioral and family therapy	1
Cognitive behavioral and interpersonal	1
CBT and medication	1
CBT, MI, DBT	1
CBT, narrative therapy	1
CBT, sex offender treatment involves polygraphs	1
Cognitive behavioral, exposure and response prevention	1
Cognitive behavioral, group	1
Cognitive behavioral, DBT, emotion focused	1
Cognitive behavioral combined with choice theory	1
Cognitive reframing helped; this involved writing the stories and discussing the rich creativity	1
Cognitive restructuring	2
Cognitive restructuring of thinking errors and treatment of underlying emotional disturbance	1
Cognitive behavioral	2
Cognitive behavioral	2
CBT that focuses on accountability	1
Cognitive behavioral, existential, mindfulness based	1
Cognitive, awareness, exposure therapy, involve the clergy and law enforcement	1
Cognitive with emphasis on consequences	1
Cognitive behavioral	1
Cognitive Behavioral	1
Combination of relationship-based and consequences	1
Compassionate, acceptance	1
Confrontation and exploration of personal factors—how it impacts life and why they do it	1

(continues)

Responses	Frequency
Confrontational and psychodynamic	1
Constant challenging of statements that are lies	1
Counseling	2
Court-ordered ones, maybe	1
DBT or similar	1
DBT	2
DBT	4
DBT, ACT	1
DBT, ACT, CBT	1
DBT, CBT to lower anxiety, cognitive retraining similar to ADHD treatment	1
DBT, cognitive	1
DBT, DBT	1
DBT, interpersonal techniques, ERP for resisting the urge, like OCD compulsions	1
DBT; relationally-based interventions	1
DBT/CBT	1
Define pathological lying	1
Depends on the individual and comorbidities	1
Depends on the presentation	1
Depends on the source of the pathology	1
Depends on underlying issues	1
Depends on underlying reasons—e.g., neglect, abuse, personality disorder	1
DBT	1
DBT	1
DBT	1
DBT	1
DBT	1
DBT	1
Don't know	3
Don't know	1
Dynamic/interpersonal, multicultural approach along with Motivational interviewing and/or DBT	1
ECT? (joke) seriously, I don't know the literature regarding treatments for lying	1
Emotion-focused treatments	1

(continues)

Responses	Frequency
Emotion-focused, interpersonal, trauma informed	1
Emotion-focused/trauma informed	1
Empathy, helping patient see the defensive functions that lying might provide	1
Family or group therapy, understanding their youth and influences	1
Family therapy, insight oriented therapy models, directness from therapist	1
Finding out motivation for compulsively lying and work on those (behavioral?)	1
Functional analysis and CBT	1
Group and individual therapy with EMDR	1
Honest confrontation of behavior and exploration of genesis/coping style	1
I am not aware of any	1
I am unsure; perhaps ACT	1
I do not know	1
I do not know	1
I don't know	1
I don't know; I see the behavior as part of antisocial or narcissistic personality	1
I don't know; I tend to view things from a behavioral lens and would want to know the function	1
I don't think it is treatable	1
I have little optimism that any intervention will succeed with people who meet the above description	1
I have no knowledge of the research	1
I think it is usually a feature or symptom of a larger problem, such as an Axis II [disorder]	1
I wish I knew	1
Identification and consequences	1
Identify ego state age equivalencies, treat via EMDR and DNMS	1
I don't know	1
Increase insight into reasons for lying (narcissism?) and negative consequences; possibly CBT	1
Insight and behavior-change interventions	1
Insight-oriented and CBT and MI	1
Insight oriented; attachment	1
Integrationist	1
Internal family systems	1
Interpersonal	1

(continues)

Responses	Frequency
Interpersonal therapy	1
Interpersonal/psychodynamic	1
Interpersonal/psychodynamic therapy, but honestly pathological lying in adulthood is not treatable	1
It depends on the personality disorder that underpins the lying	1
It depends on what other issues they have and what their own treatment goals are	1
It is likely a personality disorder and not really amenable to treatment	1
It's a form of resistance; true, may be due to anxiety/avoidance, which can be treated; otherwise no	1
Jail (sociopaths), CBT	1
Limit-setting, validation conditions, verbal praise	1
Long-term therapy with a goal of discerning the reasons for the pathological lying, as they vary	1
Long term, in-depth with a strong therapeutic relationship, simple confrontation as a technique	1
Maybe a cognitive-behavioral approach: reframe their beliefs contributing to compulsive lying	1
Moral reconditioning, antisocial psychoeducation	1
Most likely cognitive, but there may be effective behavioral strategies as well	1
MI	1
MI	1
MI, CBT	1
MI, CBT exposure, family/couples work to discuss the impact of behavior	1
N/A	1
No idea	1
None	2
Not sure	2
Not sure there is effective treatment for a willful intent to deceive people	1
Not sure	1
Not sure; think it's found across different *DSM/ICD* disorders	1
Person-centered, CBT/DBT	1
Possible social skills training, teach self-monitoring, positive behavior reinforcement	1
Possibly group therapy	1
Probably none unless the client is motivated to change	1
Psychoanalytic psychotherapy, psychoanalysis	1

(continues)

Responses	Frequency
Psychodynamic exploration	1
Psychodynamic psychotherapy, group	1
Psychodynamic psychotherapy; focus on attachment and relationship dynamics	1
Psychodynamic therapy, schema therapy, CBT	1
Psychodynamic therapy/insight-oriented therapy	1
Psychodynamic with cognitive strategies	1
Psychotherapy	1
Psychotherapy	2
Psychotherapy, hypnotherapy	1
Psychotherapy, reality therapy,	1
PTSD	1
Reality-based feedback/confrontation when identifiable	1
Reality therapy	1
Reality therapy	1
Reality Therapy	3
REBT	2
REBT, experiential feedback	1
Recovery oriented/relational confrontation	1
Reinforcement for truth-telling	1
Rogerian therapy, MI, CBT	1
Same type of treatment for OCD	1
Seeing the lying as a symptom rather than primary issue	1
Self-checks and behav. reminders (i.e., snap rubber band on wrist when lying with reward for truths)	1
Some type of reality therapy? Has to have accountability piece	1
Spiritual awakening	1
Target the person's beliefs and how those fuel the lying, then work to change the beliefs/behavior	1
The same as for any personality disorder because this is mostly the main issue with liars	1
Therapy and maybe medication	1
Therapy to examine the need for lying and provide methods to address that need other than lying	1
Therapy—CBT, ACT	1
There is no treatment	1

(*continues*)

Responses	Frequency
Thought stopping and other cognitive techniques	1
Thought/lie charts	1
Trauma-focused therapy	1
Trauma informed, DBT, ACT, CBT	1
Treatment aimed at personality makeup and CBT related to perceptions and understanding of consequences	1
Treatment recommendations would vary depending on the nature of the underlying psychopathology	1
Treatments designed to address the patterns described above	1
Unless the person is distressed by the behavior, none	1
Unsure	1
Unsure	1
Total	264

Note. ACT = acceptance and commitment therapy; ADHD = attention-deficit/hyperactivity disorder; CBT = cognitive behavior therapy; DBT = dialectical behavior therapy; DNMS = developmental needs meeting strategy; *DSM = Diagnostic and Statistical Manual of Mental Disorders*; ECT = electroconvulsive therapy; EMDR = eye-movement desensitization and reprocessing; ERP = exposure and response prevention; *ICD = International Classification of Diseases*; MI = motivational interviewing; N/A = not applicable; OCD = obsessive-compulsive disorder; PTSD = posttraumatic stress disorder; RBT = rational behavior therapy; REBT = rational emotive behavior therapy.

References

Ackert, L., Church, B., Kuang, X., & Qi, L. (2011). Lying: An experimental investigation of the role of situational factors. *Business Ethics Quarterly, 21*(4), 605–632. https://doi.org/10.5840/beq201121438

Aghababaei, N., Mohammadtabar, S., & Saffarinia, M. (2014). Dirty dozen vs. the H factor: Comparison of the dark triad and honesty–humility in prosociality, religiosity, and happiness. *Personality and Individual Differences, 67*, 6–10. https://doi.org/10.1016/j.paid.2014.03.026

Alloway, T. P., McCallum, F., Alloway, R. G., & Hoicka, E. (2015). Liar, liar, working memory on fire: Investigating the role of working memory in childhood verbal deception. *Journal of Experimental Child Psychology, 137*, 30–38. https://doi.org/10.1016/j.jecp.2015.03.013

American Psychiatric Association. (1952). *Diagnostic and statistical manual of mental disorders.* American Psychiatric Association.

American Psychiatric Association. (1987). *Diagnostic and statistical manual of mental disorders* (3rd ed.). American Psychiatric Association.

American Psychiatric Association. (1994). *Diagnostic and statistical manual of mental disorders* (4th ed.). American Psychiatric Association.

American Psychiatric Association. (2013). *Diagnostic and statistical manual of mental disorders* (5th ed.). American Psychiatric Association.

American Psychiatric Association. (2021). *Submit proposals for making changes to DSM-5.* https://www.psychiatry.org/psychiatrists/practice/dsm/submit-proposals

American Psychological Association. (2020a). *APA dictionary of psychology.* https://dictionary.apa.org/

American Psychological Association. (2020b). *APA Guidelines for Psychological Assessment and Evaluation.* https://www.apa.org/about/policy/guidelines-psychological-assessment-evaluation.pdf

American Psychological Association, Division 12. (2016). *Psychological treatments*. https://div12.org/treatments/

American Psychological Association, Presidential Task Force on Evidence-Based Practice. (2006). Evidence-based practice in psychology. *American Psychologist, 61*(4), 271–285. https://doi.org/10.1037/0003-066X.61.4.271

Anderson, D. R., Field, D. E., Collins, P. A., Lorch, E. P., & Nathan, J. G. (1985). Estimates of young children's time with television: A methodological comparison of parent reports with time-lapse video home observation. *Child Development, 56*(5), 1345–1357. https://doi.org/10.2307/1130249

Anderson, N. H. (1968). Likableness ratings of 555 personality-trait words. *Journal of Personality and Social Psychology, 9*(3), 272–279. https://doi.org/10.1037/h0025907

Apicella, C. L., Marlowe, F. W., Fowler, J. H., & Christakis, N. A. (2012). Social networks and cooperation in hunter-gatherers. *Nature, 481*(7382), 497–501. https://doi.org/10.1038/nature10736

Aquinas, T. (1947). Question 145: Of honesty (Fathers of the English Dominican Province, Trans.) in *The Summa Theologica*. Benziger Bros. (Original work published in 1485) https://www.ccel.org/a/aquinas/summa/SS/SS145.html#SSQ145OUTP1

Ariely, D. (2012). *The honest truth about dishonesty: How we lie to everyone—Especially ourselves*. HarperCollins.

Aristotle. (1941a). *Nicomachean ethics* (W. D. Ross, Trans.). In R. McKeon (Ed.), *The basic works of Aristotle* (pp. 927–1112). Random House.

Aristotle. (1941b). *Organon*. In R. McKeon (Ed.), *The basic words of Aristotle* (pp. 1–217). Random House.

Asher, R. (1951). Munchausen's syndrome. *Lancet, 257*(6650), 339–341. https://doi.org/10.1016/S0140-6736(51)92313-6

Ashton, M. C., & Lee, K. (2007). Empirical, theoretical, and practical advantages of the HEXACO model of personality structure. *Personality and Social Psychology Review, 11*(2), 150–166. https://doi.org/10.1177/1088868306294907

Ashton, M. C., & Lee, K. (2008). The HEXACO model of personality structure and the importance of the H factor. *Social and Personality Psychology Compass, 2*(5), 1952–1962. https://doi.org/10.1111/j.1751-9004.2008.00134.x

Ashton, M. C., & Lee, K. (2009). The HEXACO-60: A short measure of the major dimensions of personality. *Journal of Personality Assessment, 91*(4), 340–345. https://doi.org/10.1080/00223890902935878

Ashton, M. C., Lee, K., Perugini, M., Szarota, P., de Vries, R. E., Di Blas, L., Boies, K., & De Raad, B. (2004). A six-factor structure of personality-descriptive adjectives: Solutions from psycholexical studies in seven languages. *Journal of Personality and Social Psychology, 86*(2), 356–366. https://doi.org/10.1037/0022-3514.86.2.356

Bandura, A., Ross, D., & Ross, S. A. (1961). Transmission of aggression through imitation of aggressive models. *Journal of Abnormal and Social Psychology, 63*(3), 575–582. https://doi.org/10.1037/h0045925

Barnes, C. M., Schaubroeck, J., Huth, M., & Ghumman, S. (2011). Lack of sleep and unethical conduct. *Organizational Behavior and Human Decision Processes, 115*(2), 169–180. https://doi.org/10.1016/j.obhdp.2011.01.009

Barnett, J. E. (2011). Learning from lies at the therapist's school of hard knocks. In J. Kottler & J. Carlson (Eds.), *Duped: Lies and deception in psychotherapy* (pp. 121–126). Routledge/Taylor & Francis Group.

Bartlett, F. C. (1932). *Remembering.* Cambridge University Press.

Barton, L. E., Brulle, A. R., & Repp, A. C. (1986). Maintenance of therapeutic change by momentary DRO. *Journal of Applied Behavior Analysis, 19*(3), 277–282. https://doi.org/10.1901/jaba.1986.19-277

Bate, K. S., Malouff, J. M., Thorsteinsson, E. T., & Bhullar, N. (2011). The efficacy of habit reversal therapy for tics, habit disorders, and stuttering: A meta-analytic review. *Clinical Psychology Review, 31*(5), 865–871. https://doi.org/10.1016/j.cpr.2011.03.013

Batterham, P. J., Sunderland, M., Carragher, N., Calear, A. L., Mackinnon, A. J., & Slade, T. (2016). The Distress Questionnaire—5: Population screener for psychological distress was more accurate than the K6/K10. *Journal of Clinical Epidemiology, 71*, 35–42. https://doi.org/10.1016/j.jclinepi.2015.10.005

Baumeister, R. F., Bratslavsky, E., Muraven, M., & Tice, D. M. (1998). Ego depletion: Is the active self a limited resource? *Journal of Personality and Social Psychology, 74*(5), 1252–1265. https://doi.org/10.1037/0022-3514.74.5.1252

Baumrind, D. (1985). Research using intentional deception. Ethical issues revisited. *American Psychologist, 40*(2), 165–174. https://doi.org/10.1037/0003-066X.40.2.165

Beck, J. S. (2021). *Cognitive behavior therapy: Basics and beyond* (3rd ed.). Guilford Press.

Beech, R. M., Duncan, R., Hart, C. L., & Curtis, D. A. (2021, September). *Self-reported experiences with pathological liars.* Presented at the annual meeting of the Society for Police and Criminal Psychology, Arlington, TX.

Benjamin, L. T., Jr., & Baker, D. B. (2004). *From séance to science: A history of the profession of psychology in America.* Wadsworth/Thomson Learning.

Benning, S. D., Venables, N. C., & Hall, J. R. (2018). Successful psychopathy. In C. J. Patrick (Ed.), *Handbook of psychopathy* (pp. 585–608). Guilford Press.

Ben-Shakhar, G., Bar-Hillel, M., & Kremnitzer, M. (2002). Trial by polygraph: Reconsidering the use of the guilty knowledge technique in court. *Law and Human Behavior, 26*(5), 527–541. https://doi.org/10.1023/A:1020204005730

Bhutta, N., Bricker, J., Chang, A. C., Dettling, L. J., Goodman, S., Hsu, J. W., Moore, K. B., Reber, S., Volz, A. H., & Windle, R. A. (2020). Changes in U.S. family finances from 2016 to 2019: Evidence from the survey of consumer finances. *Federal Reserve Bulletin, 106*(5), 1–42. https://doi.org/10.17016/bulletin.2020.106

Birch, C. D., Kelln, B. R. C., & Aquino, E. P. B. (2006). A review and case report of pseudologia fantastica. *Journal of Forensic Psychiatry & Psychology, 17*(2), 299–320. https://doi.org/10.1080/14789940500485128

Blanchard, M., & Farber, B. A. (2016). Lying in psychotherapy: Why and what clients don't tell their therapist about therapy and their relationship. *Counselling Psychology Quarterly, 29*(1), 90–112. https://doi.org/10.1080/09515070.2015.1085365

Blashfield, R. K., & Burgess, D. R. (2007). Classification provides an essential basis for organizing mental disorders. In S. O. Lilienfeld, W. T. O'Donohue, S. O. Lilienfeld, & W. T. O'Donohue (Eds.), *The great ideas of clinical science: 17 principles that every mental health professional should understand* (pp. 93–117). Routledge/Taylor & Francis Group.

Blashfield, R. K., Keeley, J. W., Flanagan, E. H., & Miles, S. R. (2014). The cycle of classification: *DSM-I* through *DSM-5. Annual Review of Clinical Psychology, 10*(1), 25–51. https://doi.org/10.1146/annurev-clinpsy-032813-153639

Bogaard, G., Meijer, E. H., Vrij, A., & Merckelbach, H. (2016). Strong, but wrong: Lay people's and police officers' beliefs about verbal and nonverbal cues to deception. *PLOS ONE, 11*(6), e0156615. https://doi.org/10.1371/journal.pone.0156615

Bogaard, G., Verschuere, B., & Meijer, E. (2021). *Centre for Policing and Security: Stop offering pseudoscience.* Preprint. https://doi.org/10.13140/RG.2.2.14479.71841

Bok, S. (1978). *Lying: Moral choice in public and private life.* Vintage Books.

Bok, S. (1999). *Lying: Moral choice in public and private life* (2nd ed.). Pantheon Books.

Bond, C. F., Jr., & DePaulo, B. M. (2006). Accuracy of deception judgments. *Personality and Social Psychology Review, 10*(3), 214–234. https://doi.org/10.1207/s15327957pspr1003_2

Bond, C. F., Jr., Howard, A. R., Hutchison, J. L., & Masip, J. (2013). Overlooking the obvious: Incentives to lie. *Basic and Applied Social Psychology, 35*(2), 212–221. https://doi.org/10.1080/01973533.2013.764302

Braun, C. M. J., Larocque, C., Daigneault, S., & Montour-Proulx, I. (1999). Mania, pseudomania, depression, and pseudodepression resulting from focal unilateral cortical lesions. *Neuropsychiatry, Neuropsychology, and Behavioral Neurology*, *12*(1), 35–51.

Brenner, P. S., & DeLamater, J. (2016). Lies, damned lies, and survey self-reports? Identity as a cause of measurement bias. *Social Psychology Quarterly*, *79*(4), 333–354. https://doi.org/10.1177/0190272516628298

Briggs, J. R. (1992). *Counselor assessments of honest and deceptive clients* (Publication No. 9236373) [Doctoral dissertation, Ball State University]. ProQuest Dissertations and Theses Global.

Brown, J., Huntley, D., Morgan, S., Dodson, K. D., & Cich, J. (2017). Confabulation: A guide for mental health professionals. *International Journal of Neurology and Neurotherapy*, *4*(2), 070. https://doi.org/10.23937/2378-3001/1410070

Buckholtz, A. (2004, August 10). Feeling the heat. *The Washington Post*. https://www.washingtonpost.com/archive/lifestyle/wellness/2004/08/10/feeling-the-heat/d06ca572-bedb-418e-a91a-f76ca0de9a71/

Buller, D. B., & Burgoon, J. K. (1996). Interpersonal deception theory. *Communication Theory*, *6*(3), 203–242. https://doi.org/10.1111/j.1468-2885.1996.tb00127.x

Buss, A. R. (1977). The trait-situation controversy and the concept of interaction. *Personality and Social Psychology Bulletin*, *3*(2), 196–201. https://doi.org/10.1177/014616727700300207

Butcher, J. N., Dahlstrom, W. G., Graham, J. R., Tellegen, A., & Kaemmer, B. (2001). *The Minnesota Multiphasic Personality Inventory-2 (MMPI-2-Revised): Manual for administration and scoring*. University of Minnesota Press.

Buzar, S., Jalšenjak, B., Krkaä, K., Lukin, J., Mladiä, D., & Spajiä, I. (2010). Habitual lying. *Philosophical Papers and Reviews*, *2*(3), 34–39.

Cargill, J. R., & Curtis, D. A. (2017). Parental deception: Perceived effects on parent–child relationships. *Journal of Relationships Research*, *8*, e1. https://doi.org/10.1017/jrr.2017.1

Carlson, J. (2011). Why I do what I do. In J. Kottler & J. Carlson (Eds.), *Duped: Lies and deception in psychotherapy* (pp. 15–19). Routledge/Taylor & Francis Group.

Childs, J. (2013). Personal characteristics and lying: An experimental investigation. *Economics Letters*, *121*(3), 425–427. https://doi.org/10.1016/j.econlet.2013.09.005

Choshen-Hillel, S., Shaw, A., & Caruso, E. M. (2020). Lying to appear honest. *Journal of Experimental Psychology: General*, *149*(9), 1719–1735. https://doi.org/10.1037/xge0000737

Clark, J. P., & Tifft, L. L. (1966). Polygraph and interview validation of self-reported deviant behavior. *American Sociological Review, 31*(4), 516–523. https://doi.org/10.2307/2090775

Clark, N. (1718). *A compleat body of divinity: Consonant to the doctrine of the Church of England.* Bible and Crown.

Cohen, T. R., Gunia, B. C., Kim-Jun, S. Y., & Murnighan, J. K. (2009). Do groups lie more than individuals? Honesty and deception as a function of strategic self-interest. *Journal of Experimental Social Psychology, 45*(6), 1321–1324. https://doi.org/10.1016/j.jesp.2009.08.007

Cohen, T. R., Meier, B. P., Hinsz, V. B., & Insko, C. A. (2010). When and why group interactions are competitive, and how competition can be replaced with cooperation. In S. Schuman (Ed.), *The handbook for working with difficult groups* (pp. 223–236). Jossey-Bass.

Cohen, T. R., Panter, A. T., & Turan, N. (2012). Guilt proneness and moral character. *Current Directions in Psychological Science, 21*(5), 355–359. https://doi.org/10.1177/0963721412454874

Cole, T. (2001). Lying to the one you love: The use of deception in romantic relationships. *Journal of Social and Personal Relationships, 18*(1), 107–129. https://doi.org/10.1177/0265407501181005

Collett, D., & Lewis, T. (1976). The subjective nature of outlier rejection procedures. *Journal of the Royal Statistical Society. Series C, Applied Statistics, 25*(3), 228–237. https://doi.org/10.2307/2347230

Conrath, D. W., Higgins, C. A., & McClean, R. J. (1983). A comparison of the reliability of questionnaire versus diary data. *Social Networks, 5*(3), 315–322. https://doi.org/10.1016/0378-8733(83)90031-X

Costa, P. T., Jr., & McCrae, R. R. (1992). *Revised NEO Personality Inventory (NEO-PI–R) and the NEO Five-Factor Inventory (NEO-FFI) professional manual.* Psychological Assessment Resources.

Covrig, C., Mateiciuc, D.-I., Radu, S.-V., & Dinca, L. A. (2013). Case study: Differential diagnosis between organic personality disorder and antisocial personality disorder. *Bulletin of Integrative Psychiatry, 19*(1), 56+. https://link.gale.com/apps/doc/A464663922/AONE?u=googlescholar&sid=bookmark-AONE&xid=5a7ab9df

Cox, D. R., & Lewis, P. A. W. (1966). *The statistical analysis of series of events.* Methuen. https://doi.org/10.1007/978-94-011-7801-3

Curtis, D. A. (2013). *Therapists' beliefs and attitudes towards client deception* (Publication No. 1508454518) [Doctoral dissertation, Texas Woman's University]. ProQuest Dissertations and Theses Global.

Curtis, D. A. (2015). Patient deception: Nursing professionals' beliefs and attitudes. *Nurse Educator*, *40*(5), 254–257. https://doi.org/10.1097/NNE. 0000000000000157

Curtis, D. A. (2019, April). *Pseudologia phantastica—Pathological lying: A theory*. Professional representative symposium presented at the 65th Annual Southwestern Psychological Association Conference, Albuquerque, NM.

Curtis, D. A. (2021a). Deception detection and emotion recognition: Investigating F.A.C.E. software. *Psychotherapy Research*, *31*(6), 802–816. https://doi.org/10.1080/10503307.2020.1836424

Curtis, D. A. (2021b). You liar! Attributions of lying. *Journal of Language and Social Psychology*, *40*(4), 504–523. https://doi.org/10.1177/0261927X21999692

Curtis, D. A., Braziel, J. M., Redfearn, R. A., & Hall, J. (2020). Lying to patients: Ethics of deception in nursing. *Clinical Ethics*, *16*(4), 341–346. https://doi.org/10.1177/1477750920977103

Curtis, D. A., & Dickens, C. (2017, March). *Myth busting: Beliefs and attitudes toward deception*. Workshop presented at the 63rd Annual Southwestern Psychological Association Conference, San Antonio, TX.

Curtis, D. A., & Hart, C. L. (2015). Does Pinocchio's nose grow in therapy? Therapists' attitudes and beliefs toward client deception. *International Journal for the Advancement of Counseling*, *37*(3), 279–292. https://doi.org/10.1007/s10447-015-9243-6

Curtis, D. A., & Hart, C. L. (2020a). Deception in psychotherapy: Frequency, typology, and relationship. *Counselling & Psychotherapy Research*, *20*(1), 106–115. https://doi.org/10.1002/capr.12263

Curtis, D. A., & Hart, C. L. (2020b). Pathological lying: Theoretical and empirical support for a diagnostic entity. *Psychiatric Research and Clinical Practice*, *2*(2), 62–69. https://doi.org/10.1176/appi.prcp.20190046

Curtis, D. A., & Hart, C. L. (2021a). *Assessment of pathological lying* [Unpublished manuscript]. Angelo State University, San Angelo, TX.

Curtis, D. A., & Hart, C. L. (2021b). *Pathological lying found in blogs, forums, and videos* [Unpublished manuscript]. Angelo State University, San Angelo, TX.

Curtis, D. A., & Hart, C. L. (2021c). Pathological lying: Psychotherapists' experiences and ability to diagnose. *American Journal of Psychotherapy*. Advance online publication. https://doi.org/10.1176/appi.psychotherapy.20210006

Curtis, D. A., Hart, C. L., & Schneemann, A. (2021). *A psycholinguistic analysis of pathological liars* [Manuscript submitted for publication]. Angelo State University, San Angelo, TX.

Curtis, D. A., Huang, H.-H., & Nicks, K. L. (2018). Patient deception in health care: Physical therapy education, beliefs, and attitudes. *International Journal of Health Sciences Education*, *5*(1). https://core.ac.uk/download/pdf/214088236.pdf

Curtis, D. A., & Kelley, L. (2016). *Abnormal psychology: Myths of "crazy."* Kendall Hunt.

Curtis, D. A., & Kelley, L. (2020a). *Abnormal psychology: Myths of "crazy"* (3rd ed.). Kendall Hunt.

Curtis, D. A., & Kelley, L. J. (2020b). Ethics of psychotherapist deception. *Ethics & Behavior, 30*(8), 601–616. https://doi.org/10.1080/10508422.2019.1674654

Curtis, D. A., & Kelley, L. J. (2021). Psychomythology of psychopathology: Myths and mythbusting in teaching abnormal psychology. *Teaching of Psychology.* Advance online publication. https://doi.org/10.1177/00986283211023195

Daiku, Y., Serota, K. B., & Levine, T. R. (2021). A few prolific liars in Japan: Replication and the effects of dark triad personality traits. *PLOS ONE, 16*(4), e0249815. https://doi.org/10.1371/journal.pone.0249815

Daubert v. Merrell Dow Pharmaceuticals, Inc., 509 U.S. 579 (1993).

Davison, G. C., & Lazarus, A. A. (2007). Clinical case studies are important in the science and practice of psychotherapy. In S. O. Lilienfeld & W. T. O'Donohue (Eds.), *The great ideas of clinical science: 17 principles that every mental health professional should understand* (pp. 149–162). Routledge/Taylor & Francis Group.

Debey, E., De Schryver, M., Logan, G. D., Suchotzki, K., & Verschuere, B. (2015). From junior to senior Pinocchio: A cross-sectional lifespan investigation of deception. *Acta Psychologica, 160*, 58–68. https://doi.org/10.1016/j.actpsy.2015.06.007

Delbrück, A. (1891). *The pathological lie and the mentally abnormal dodgers, an investigation of the gradual transition from a normal psychological process into a pathological symptom for doctors and lawyers.*

Delton, A. W., Krasnow, M. M., Cosmides, L., & Tooby, J. (2011). Evolution of direct reciprocity under uncertainty can explain human generosity in one-shot encounters. *Proceedings of the National Academy of Sciences of the United States of America, 108*(32), 13335–13340. https://doi.org/10.1073/pnas.1102131108

DePaulo, B. M., Ansfield, M. E., Kirkendol, S. E., & Boden, J. M. (2004). Serious lies. *Basic and Applied Social Psychology, 26*(2-3), 147–167. https://doi.org/10.1080/01973533.2004.9646402

DePaulo, B. M., Epstein, J. A., & Wyer, M. M. (1993). Sex differences in lying: How women and men deal with the dilemma of deceit. In M. Lewis & C. Saarni (Eds.), *Lying and deception in everyday life* (pp. 126–147). Guilford Press.

DePaulo, B. M., & Kashy, D. A. (1998). Everyday lies in close and casual relationships. *Journal of Personality and Social Psychology, 74*(1), 63–79. https://doi.org/10.1037/0022-3514.74.1.63

DePaulo, B. M., Kashy, D. A., Kirkendol, S. E., Wyer, M. M., & Epstein, J. A. (1996). Lying in everyday life. *Journal of Personality and Social Psychology, 70*(5), 979–995. https://doi.org/10.1037/0022-3514.70.5.979

DeSteno, D., Duong, F., Lim, D., & Kates, S. (2019). The grateful don't cheat: Gratitude as a fount of virtue. *Psychological Science, 30*(7), 979–988. https://doi.org/10.1177/0956797619848351

Deutsch, H., & Roazen, P. (1982). On the pathological lie (pseudologia phantastica). *The Journal of the American Academy of Psychoanalysis, 10*(3), 369–386. (Original work published in German in 1922) https://doi.org/10.1521/jaap.1.1982.10.3.369

Dewsbury, D. A. (1997). On the evolution of divisions. *The American Psychologist, 52*(7), 733–741.

Dickens, C. R., & Curtis, D. A. (2019). Lies within the law: Therapist' beliefs and attitudes about deception. *Journal of Forensic Psychology Research and Practice, 19*(5), 359–375. https://doi.org/10.1080/24732850.2019.1666604

Dike, C. C. (2008). Pathological lying: Symptom or disease? *The Psychiatric Times, 25*, 67–73.

Dike, C. C. (2020). A radical reexamination of the association between pathological lying and factitious disorder. *The Journal of the American Academy of Psychiatry and the Law, 48*(4), 431–435.

Dike, C. C., Baranoski, M., & Griffith, E. E. H. (2005). Pathological lying revisited. *The Journal of the American Academy of Psychiatry and the Law, 33*(3), 342–349.

Dimitrakopoulos, S., Sakadaki, E., & Ploumpidis, D. (2014). Pseudologia fantastica à deux: Review and case study. *Psychiatriki, 25*(3), 192–199.

Domjan, M. (2003). *The principles of learning and behavior* (5th ed.). Thomson/Wadsworth.

Drouin, M., Miller, D. A., Wehle, S., & Hernandez, E. (2016). Why do people lie online? "Because everyone lies on the internet." *Computers in Human Behavior, 64*, 134–142. https://doi.org/10.1016/j.chb.2016.06.052

Dubois, D., Rucker, D. D., & Galinsky, A. D. (2015). Social class, power, and selfishness: When and why upper and lower class individuals behave unethically. *Journal of Personality and Social Psychology, 108*(3), 436–449. https://doi.org/10.1037/pspi0000008

Dunbar, N. E., & Johnson, A. J. (2015). A test of dyadic power theory: Control attempts recalled from interpersonal interactions with romantic partners, family members, and friends. *Journal of Argumentation in Context, 4*(1), 42–62. https://doi.org/10.1075/jaic.4.1.03dun

Dupré, E. (1905). *Mythomania. Psychological and forensic study of lies and morbid storytelling.* Imprimerie typographie Jean Gainche.

Ebbinghaus, H. (1885). *Über das Gedächtnis* [About the memory]. Dunker.

Ebbinghaus, H. (1908). *Psychology: An elementary textbook.* Heath. https://doi.org/10.1037/13638-000

Edwards, B. G., Albertson, E., & Verona, E. (2017). Dark and vulnerable personality trait correlates of dimensions of criminal behavior among adult offenders.

Journal of Abnormal Psychology, 126(7), 921–927. https://doi.org/10.1037/abn0000281

Ekman, P. (1985). *Telling lies: Clues to deceit in the marketplace, politics, and marriage.* Norton & Company.

Ekman, P. (2021). *Why do people lie?* https://www.paulekman.com/blog/why-do-people-lie-motives/

Ekman, P., O'Sullivan, M., & Frank, M. G. (1999). A few can catch a liar. *Psychological Science, 10*, 263–266. https://doi.org/10.1111/1467-9280.00147

Elaad, E., & Reizer, A. (2015). Personality correlates of the self-assessed abilities to tell and detect lies, tell truths, and believe others. *Journal of Individual Differences, 36*(3), 163–169. https://doi.org/10.1027/1614-0001/a000168

Engel, G. L. (1996). From biomedical to biopsychosocial: I. Being scientific in the human domain. *Families, Systems, & Health, 14*(4), 425–433. https://doi.org/10.1037/h0089973

Ennis, E., Vrij, A., & Chance, C. (2008). Individual differences and lying in everyday life. *Journal of Social and Personal Relationships, 25*(1), 105–118. https://doi.org/10.1177/0265407507086808

Erat, S., & Gneezy, U. (2012). White lies. *Management Science, 58*(4), 723–733. https://doi.org/10.1287/mnsc.1110.1449

Esteves, G. G. L., Oliveira, L. S., Andrade, J. M., & Menezes, M. P. (2021). Dark triad predicts academic cheating. *Personality and Individual Differences, 171*, 110513. https://doi.org/10.1016/j.paid.2020.110513

Eswara, H. S., & Suryarekha, A. (1974). The relationship between lie scores and anxiety scores on Taylor's Manifest Anxiety Scale. *Journal of Psychological Researches, 18*(3), 88–90.

Fallowfield, L. J., Jenkins, V. A., & Beveridge, H. A. (2002). Truth may hurt but deceit hurts more: Communication in palliative care. *Palliative Medicine, 16*(4), 297–303. https://doi.org/10.1191/0269216302pm575oa

Farber, B., Blanchard, M., & Love, M. (2019). *Secrets and lies in psychotherapy.* American Psychological Association. https://doi.org/10.1037/0000128-000

Farhat, L. C., Olfson, E., Nasir, M., Levine, J. L. S., Li, F., Miguel, E. C., & Bloch, M. H. (2020). Pharmacological and behavioral treatment for trichotillomania: An updated systematic review with meta-analysis. *Depression & Anxiety, 37*(8), 715–727. https://doi.org/10.1002/da.23028

Feldman, R. S., Forrest, J. A., & Happ, B. R. (2002). Self-presentation and verbal deception: Do self-presenters lie more? *Basic and Applied Social Psychology, 24*(2), 163–170. https://doi.org/10.1207/S15324834BASP2402_8

Fellner, G., Sausgruber, R., & Traxler, C. (2013). Testing enforcement strategies in the field: Threat, moral appeal and social information. *Journal of the European Economic Association, 11*(3), 634–660. https://doi.org/10.1111/jeea.12013

Festinger, L. (1957). *A theory of cognitive dissonance*. Stanford University Press.

Figee, M., Pattij, T., Willuhn, I., Luigjes, J., van den Brink, W., Goudriaan, A., Potenza, M. N., Robbins, T. W., & Denys, D. (2016). Compulsivity in obsessive-compulsive disorder and addictions. *European Neuropsychopharmacology: The Journal of the European College of Neuropsychopharmacology, 26*(5), 856–868. https://doi.org/10.1016/j.euroneuro.2015.12.003

Flexon, J. L., Meldrum, R. C., Young, J. T. N., & Lehmann, P. S. (2016). Low self-control and the Dark Triad: Disentangling the predictive power of personality traits on young adult substance use, offending and victimization. *Journal of Criminal Justice, 46*, 159–169. https://doi.org/10.1016/j.jcrimjus.2016.05.006

Floch, M. (1950). Limitations of the lie detector. *Journal of Criminal Law & Criminology (08852731), 40*(5), 651–653.

Foerster, A., Pfister, R., Schmidts, C., Dignath, D., & Kunde, W. (2013). Honesty saves time (and justifications). *Frontiers in Psychology, 4*, 473. https://doi.org/10.3389/fpsyg.2013.00473

Ford, C. V. (1996). *Lies! Lies!! Lies!!!: The psychology of deceit*. American Psychiatric Association.

Ford, C. V., King, B. H., & Hollender, M. H. (1988). Lies and liars: Psychiatric aspects of prevarication. *The American Journal of Psychiatry, 145*(5), 554–562. https://doi.org/10.1176/ajp.145.5.554

Frances, A. (2013). *Saving normal: An insider's revolt against out-of-control psychiatric diagnosis, DSM-5, big pharma, and the medicalization of ordinary life*. William Morrow.

Franklin, B. (1750). *Poor Richard's improved almanack*. New Printing Office.

Frierson, R. L., & Joshi, K. G. (2018). Implications of pseudologia fantastica in criminal forensic evaluations: A review and case report. *Journal of Forensic Sciences, 63*(3), 976–979. https://doi.org/10.1111/1556-4029.13616

Ganis, G. (2015). Deception detection using neuroimaging. In P. A. Granhag, A. Vrij, & B. Verschuere (Eds.), *Detecting deception: Current challenges and cognitive approaches* (pp. 105–121). Wiley-Blackwell.

Gardner, W., Mulvey, E. P., & Shaw, E. C. (1995). Regression analyses of counts and rates: Poisson, overdispersed Poisson, and negative binomial models. *Psychological Bulletin, 118*(3), 392–404. https://doi.org/10.1037/0033-2909.118.3.392

Garlipp, P. (2017). Pseudologia fantastica—Pathological lying. In B. A. Sharpless (Ed.), *Unusual and rare psychological disorders: A handbook for clinical practice and research* (pp. 319–327). Oxford University Press. https://doi.org/10.1093/med:psych/9780190245863.001.0001

George, J., & Robb, A. (2008). Deception and computer-mediated communication in daily life. *Communication Reports, 21*(2), 92–103. https://doi.org/10.1080/08934210802298108

Gerlach, P., Teodorescu, K., & Hertwig, R. (2019). The truth about lies: A meta-analysis on dishonest behavior. *Psychological Bulletin, 145*(1), 1–44. https://doi.org/10.1037/bul0000174

Gervais, W. M., Shariff, A. F., & Norenzayan, A. (2011). Do you believe in atheists? Distrust is central to anti-atheist prejudice. *Journal of Personality and Social Psychology, 101*(6), 1189–1206. https://doi.org/10.1037/a0025882

Gillard, N. D. (2018). Psychopathy and deception. In R. Rogers & S. D. Bender (Eds.), *Clinical assessment of malingering and deception* (pp. 174–187). Guilford Press.

Gino, F., & Ariely, D. (2012). The dark side of creativity: Original thinkers can be more dishonest. *Journal of Personality and Social Psychology, 102*(3), 445–459. https://doi.org/10.1037/a0026406

Gino, F., & Galinsky, A. D. (2012). Vicarious dishonesty: When psychological closeness creates distance from one's moral compass. *Organizational Behavior and Human Decision Processes, 119*(1), 15–26. https://doi.org/10.1016/j.obhdp.2012.03.011

Gino, F., & Mogilner, C. (2014). Time, money, and morality. *Psychological Science, 25*(2), 414–421. https://doi.org/10.1177/0956797613506438

Gino, F., Schweitzer, M. E., Mead, N. L., & Ariely, D. (2011). Unable to resist temptation: How self-control depletion promotes unethical behavior. *Organizational Behavior and Human Decision Processes, 115*(2), 191–203. https://doi.org/10.1016/j.obhdp.2011.03.001

Glätzle-Rützler, D., & Lergetporer, P. (2015). Lying and age: An experimental study. *Journal of Economic Psychology, 46*, 12–25. https://doi.org/10.1016/j.joep.2014.11.002

Global Deception Research Team. (2006). A world of lies. *Journal of Cross-Cultural Psychology, 37*(1), 60–74. https://doi.org/10.1177/0022022105282295

Gneezy, U. (2005). Deception: The role of consequences. *The American Economic Review, 95*(1), 384–394. https://doi.org/10.1257/0002828053828662

Gneezy, U., Kajackaite, A., & Sobel, J. (2018). Lying aversion and the size of the lie. *The American Economic Review, 108*(2), 419–453. https://doi.org/10.1257/aer.20161553

Gogineni, R. R., & Newmark, T. (2014). Pseudologia fantastica: A fascinating case report. *Psychiatric Annals, 44*(10), 451–454. https://doi.org/10.3928/00485713-20141003-02

Granhag, P. A., & Strömwall, L. A. (2004). *The detection of deception in forensic contexts.* Cambridge University Press. https://doi.org/10.1017/CBO9780511490071

Granhag, P. A., Vrij, A., & Verschuere, B. (2015). *Detecting deception: Current challenges and cognitive approaches.* Wiley-Blackwell.

Grant, J. E., Paglia, H. A., & Chamberlain, S. R. (2019). The phenomenology of lying in young adults and relationships with personality and cognition. *Psychiatric Quarterly, 90*(2), 361–369. https://doi.org/10.1007/s11126-018-9623-2

Green, G. S. (1990). Resurrecting polygraph validation of self-reported crime data: A note on research method and ethics using the deer poacher. *Deviant Behavior, 11*(2), 131–137. https://doi.org/10.1080/01639625.1990.9967838

Green, H., James, R. A., Gilbert, J. D., & Byard, R. W. (1999). Medicolegal complications of pseudologia fantastica. *Legal Medicine, 1*(4), 254–256. https://doi.org/10.1016/S1344-6223(99)80046-7

Greene, R. L. (2011). *The MMPI-2/MMPI-2-RF: An interpretive manual* (3rd ed.). Allyn & Bacon.

Gross, A., Farrar, M. J., & Liner, D. (1982). Reduction of trichotillomania in a retarded cerebral palsied child using overcorrection, facial screening, and differential reinforcement of other behavior. *Education & Treatment of Children, 5*(2), 133–140.

Gross, C. G. (1999). A hole in the head. *The Neuroscientist, 5*(4), 263–269. https://doi.org/10.1177/107385849900500415

Groth-Marnat, G., & Wright, A. J. (2016). *Handbook of psychological assessment* (6th ed.). John Wiley & Sons, Inc.

Grzegorek, J. L. (2011). Smoke and mirrors. In J. Kottler & J. Carlson (Eds.), *Duped: Lies and deception in psychotherapy* (pp. 33–37). Routledge/Taylor & Francis Group.

Halevy, R., Shalvi, S., & Verschuere, B. (2014). Being honest about dishonesty: Correlating self-reports and actual lying. *Human Communication Research, 40*(1), 54–72. https://doi.org/10.1111/hcre.12019

Hall, G. S. (1890). Children's lies. *The American Journal of Psychology, 3*(1), 59–70. https://doi.org/10.2307/1411497

Hancock, J. T., Thom-Santelli, J., & Ritchie, T. (2004). Deception and design: The impact of communication technology on lying behavior. *CHI '04: Proceedings of the SIGCHI Conference on Human Factors in Computing Systems* (pp. 129–134). https://doi.org/10.1145/985692.985709

Hardie, T. J., & Reed, A. (1998). Pseudologia fantastica, factitious disorder and impostership: A deception syndrome. *Medicine, Science, and the Law, 38*(3), 198–201. https://doi.org/10.1177/002580249803800303

Hare, R. D. (1991). *Manual for the Revised Psychopathy Checklist.* Multi-Health Systems.

Hare, R. D. (1996). Psychopathy and antisocial personality disorder: A case of diagnostic confusion. *The Psychiatric Times, 13*(2), 39–40.

Hare, R. D. (1999). *Without conscience: The disturbing world of the psychopaths among us.* Guilford Press.

Harrigan, J. A., Kues, J. R., Steffen, J. J., & Rosenthal, R. (1987). Self-touching and impressions of others. *Personality and Social Psychology Bulletin, 13*(4), 497–512. https://doi.org/10.1177/0146167287134007

Harris, S. (2013). *Lying*. Four Elephants Press.

Hart, C., Jones, J., Terrizzi, J., & Curtis, D. (2019). Development of the Lying in Everyday Situations Scale. *The American Journal of Psychology, 132*(3), 343–352. https://doi.org/10.5406/amerjpsyc.132.3.0343

Hart, C. L. (2019). What is a lie? Defining different elements of dishonesty. *Psychology Today*. https://www.psychologytoday.com/us/blog/the-nature-deception/201905/what-is-lie

Hart, C. L., Beech, R., & Curtis, D. A. (2022). *Experiences with pathological liars* [Manuscript in preparation]. Department of Psychology & Philosophy, Texas Woman's University.

Hart, C. L., & Curtis, D. A. (in press). *Big liars: How pathological and compulsive deceivers hurt, gaslight, and exasperate everyone around them*. American Psychological Association.

Hart, C. L., Curtis, D. A., & Randell, J. A. (2022). *Pathological Lying Inventory*. Human Deception Laboratory. https://christianlhart.com/pli

Hart, C. L., Curtis, D. A., Williams, N. M., Hathaway, M. D., & Griffith, J. D. (2014). Do as I say, not as I do: Benevolent deception in romantic relationships. *Journal of Relationships Research, 5*, e8. https://doi.org/10.1017/jrr.2014.8

Hartwig, M., Granhag, P. A., Strömwall, L. A., & Kronkvist, O. (2006). Strategic use of evidence during police interviews: When training to detect deception works. *Law and Human Behavior, 30*(5), 603–619. https://doi.org/10.1007/s10979-006-9053-9

Hartwig, M., Granhag, P. A., Strömwall, L. A., & Vrij, A. (2005). Detecting deception via strategic disclosure of evidence. *Law and Human Behavior, 29*(4), 469–484. https://doi.org/10.1007/s10979-005-5521-x

Haw, C., & Stubbs, J. (2010). Covert administration of medication to older adults: A review of the literature and published studies. *Journal of Psychiatric and Mental Health Nursing, 17*(9), 761–768. https://doi.org/10.1111/j.1365-2850.2010.01613.x

Hazan, C., & Shaver, P. R. (1994). Attachment as an organizational framework for research on close relationships. *Psychological Inquiry, 5*(1), 1–22. https://doi.org/10.1207/s15327965pli0501_1

Healy, W., & Healy, M. T. (1915). Pathological lying, accusation and swindling. *Criminal Science Monographs, 1*, 1–278.

Heck, D. W., Thielmann, I., Moshagen, M., & Hilbig, B. E. (2018). Who lies? A large-scale reanalysis linking basic personality traits to unethical decision making. *Judgment and Decision Making, 13*(4), 356–371. https://journal.sjdm.org/18/18322/jdm18322.html

Heintz, C., Karabegovic, M., & Molnar, A. (2016). The co-evolution of honesty and strategic vigilance. *Frontiers in Psychology, 7*, 1503. https://doi.org/10.3389/fpsyg.2016.01503

Helm, K. (2011). Grateful for the lessons learned. In J. Kottler & J. Carlson (Eds.), *Duped: Lies and deception in psychotherapy* (pp. 79–83). Routledge/Taylor & Francis Group.

Heyman, G. D., Luu, D. H., & Lee, K. (2009). Parenting by lying. *Journal of Moral Education, 38*(3), 353–369. https://doi.org/10.1080/03057240903101630

Himle, M. B., Woods, D. W., Piacentini, J. C., & Walkup, J. T. (2006). Brief review of habit reversal training for Tourette syndrome. *Journal of Child Neurology, 21*(8), 719–725. https://doi.org/10.1177/08830738060210080101

Hirst, E. S. J., Lockenour, F. M., & Allen, J. L. (2019). Decreasing toe walking with differential reinforcement of other behavior, verbal rules, and feedback. *Education & Treatment of Children, 42*(2), 185–199. https://doi.org/10.1353/etc.2019.0009

Hofmann, W., Wisneski, D. C., Brandt, M. J., & Skitka, L. J. (2014). Morality in everyday life. *Science, 345*(6202), 1340–1343. https://doi.org/10.1126/science.1251560

Hollender, M. H., & Hersh, S. P. (1970). Impossible consultation made possible. *Archives of General Psychiatry, 23*(4), 343–345. https://doi.org/10.1001/archpsyc.1970.01750040055008

Humintell. (2020). *About us.* https://www.humintell.com/about-us/

Iacono, W. G., & Patrick, C. J. (2018). Assessing deception: Polygraph techniques and integrity testing. In R. Rogers & S. D. Bender (Eds.), *Clinical assessment of malingering and deception* (4th ed., pp. 361–386). Guilford Press.

Jackson, J. C. (2001). *Truth, trust and medicine.* Routledge.

James, W. (1890). *The principles of psychology.* Henry Holt & Co.

Jaspers, K. (1963). *General psychopathology* (7th ed.; J. Hoenig & M. H. Hamilton, Trans.). Manchester University Press. (Original work published 1913)

Jensen, L. A., Arnett, J. J., Feldman, S. S., & Cauffman, E. (2004). The right to do wrong: Lying to parents among adolescents and emerging adults. *Journal of Youth and Adolescence, 33*(2), 101–112. https://doi.org/10.1023/B:JOYO.0000013422.48100.5a

Jonason, P. K., Lyons, M., Baughman, H. M., & Vernon, P. A. (2014). What a tangled web we weave: The dark triad traits and deception. *Personality and Individual Differences, 70*, 117–119. https://doi.org/10.1016/j.paid.2014.06.038

Kalish, N. (2004). How honest are you? *Reader's Digest, 164*(981), 114–119.

Kant, I. (1996). On a supposed right to lie from philanthropy. In M. Gregor (Ed.), *The Cambridge edition of the works of Immanuel Kant: Practical philosophy* (pp. 605–616). Cambridge University Press. (Original work published 1797)

Kashy, D. A., & DePaulo, B. M. (1996). Who lies? *Journal of Personality and Social Psychology, 70*(5), 1037–1051. https://doi.org/10.1037/0022-3514.70.5.1037

Kellerman, H. (2009). *Dictionary of psychopathology.* Columbia University Press. https://doi.org/10.7312/kell14650

Kenrick, D. T., & Funder, D. C. (1988). Profiting from controversy. Lessons from the person–situation debate. *American Psychologist, 43*(1), 23–34. https://doi.org/10.1037/0003-066X.43.1.23

King, B. H., & Ford, C. V. (1988). Pseudologia fantastica. *Acta Psychiatrica Scandinavica, 77*(1), 1–6. https://doi.org/10.1111/j.1600-0447.1988.tb05068.x

King, L. W. (2008). *The code of Hammurabi.* https://avalon.law.yale.edu/ancient/hamframe.asp

Kocher, M. G., Schudy, S., & Spantig, L. (2018). I lie? We lie! Why? Experimental evidence on a dishonesty shift in groups. *Management Science, 64*(9), 3995–4008. https://doi.org/10.1287/mnsc.2017.2800

Konnikova, M. (2016). *The confidence game: Why we fall for it . . . every time.* Penguin.

Köppen, M. (1898). Ueber die pathologische Luge (Pseudo-logia phantastica) [About the pathological lie (Pseudo-logia phantastica)]. *Charite-Annalen, 8,* 674–719.

Korenis, P., Gonzalez, L., Kadriu, B., Tyagi, A., & Udolisa, A. (2015). Pseudologia fantastica: Forensic and clinical treatment implications. *Comprehensive Psychiatry, 56,* 17–20. https://doi.org/10.1016/j.comppsych.2014.09.009

Korkeila, J. A., Martin, T. E., Taiminen, T. J., Heinimaa, M., & Vourinen, E. (1995). Clarification of pseudologia fantastica: A study of two cases of fantastic pseudology. *Nordic Journal of Psychiatry, 49*(5), 367–371. https://doi.org/10.3109/08039489509011929

Kottler, J., & Carlson, J. (2011). *Duped: Lies and deception in psychotherapy.* Routledge/Taylor & Francis Group.

Kouchaki, M., & Smith, I. H. (2014). The morning morality effect: The influence of time of day on unethical behavior. *Psychological Science, 25*(1), 95–102. https://doi.org/10.1177/0956797613498099

Kowalski, R. M., Walker, S., Wilkinson, R., Queen, A., & Sharpe, B. (2003). Lying, cheating, complaining, and other aversive interpersonal behaviors: A narrative examination of the darker side of relationships. *Journal of Social and Personal Relationships, 20*(4), 471–490. https://doi.org/10.1177/02654075030204003

Kraepelin, E. (1912). *Clinical psychiatry: A textbook for students and physicians.* MacMillan. (Original work published 1902)

Kraepelin, E. (1919/1971). *Dementia praecox and paraphrenia* (R. M. Barclay, Trans.) Robert E. Krieger Publishing Co.

Kramer, S. R., & Shariff, A. F. (2016). Religion, deception, and self-deception. In J.-W. van Prooijen & P. A. M. van Lange (Eds.), *Cheating, corruption, and concealment: The roots of dishonesty* (pp. 233–249). Cambridge University Press.

Kwok, Y. L., Gralton, J., & McLaws, M. L. (2015). Face touching: A frequent habit that has implications for hand hygiene. *American Journal of Infection Control, 43*(2), 112–114. https://doi.org/10.1016/j.ajic.2014.10.015

Laland, K. (2017). On the origin of cooperation. *New Atlantis, 52,* 70–85. https://www.jstor.org/stable/44252651

Lavi, N., & Friesem, D. E. (2019). *Towards a broader view of hunter-gatherer sharing.* https://doi.org/10.17863/CAM.47185

Lavoie, J., Leduc, K., Arruda, C., Crossman, A. M., & Talwar, V. (2017). Developmental profiles of children's spontaneous lie-telling behavior. *Cognitive Development, 41,* 33–45. https://doi.org/10.1016/j.cogdev.2016.12.002

Lavoie, J., Yachison, S., Crossman, A., & Talwar, V. (2017). Polite, instrumental, and dual liars: Relation to children's developing social skills and cognitive ability. *International Journal of Behavioral Development, 41*(2), 257–264. https://doi.org/10.1177/0165025415626518

Leduc, K., Williams, S., Gomez-Garibello, C., & Talwar, V. (2017). The contributions of mental state understanding and executive functioning to preschool-aged children's lie-telling. *British Journal of Developmental Psychology, 35*(2), 288–302. https://doi.org/10.1111/bjdp.12163

Lee, K. (2000). The development of lying: How children do deceptive things with words. In J. W. Astington (Ed.), *Minds in the making* (pp. 177–196). Blackwell.

Lee, K., Talwar, V., McCarthy, A., Ross, I., Evans, A., & Arruda, C. (2014). Can classic moral stories promote honesty in children? *Psychological Science, 25*(8), 1630–1636. https://doi.org/10.1177/0956797614536401

Leventhal, B. L. (2012). Lumpers and splitters: Who knows? Who cares? *Journal of the American Academy of Child & Adolescent Psychiatry, 51*(1), 6–7. https://doi.org/10.1016/j.jaac.2011.10.009

Levine, E. E., & Schweitzer, M. E. (2014). Are liars ethical? On the tension between benevolence and honesty. *Journal of Experimental Social Psychology, 53,* 107–117. https://doi.org/10.1016/j.jesp.2014.03.005

Levine, E. E., & Schweitzer, M. E. (2015). Prosocial lies: When deception breeds trust. *Organizational Behavior and Human Decision Processes, 126,* 88–106. https://doi.org/10.1016/j.obhdp.2014.10.007

Levine, T. R. (2014a). *Encyclopedia of deception.* Sage Publications. https://doi.org/10.4135/9781483306902

Levine, T. R. (2014b). Truth-default theory (TDT): A theory of human deception and deception detection. *Journal of Language and Social Psychology, 33*(4), 378–392. https://doi.org/10.1177/0261927X14535916

Levine, T. R. (2020). *Duped: Truth-default theory and the social science of lying and deception.* University Alabama Press.

Levine, T. R., Ali, M. V., Dean, M., Abdulla, R. A., & Garcia-Ruano, K. (2016). Toward a pan-cultural typology of deception motives. *Journal of Intercultural Communication Research, 45*(1), 1–12. https://doi.org/10.1080/17475759.2015.1137079

Levine, T. R., Clare, D. D., Blair, J. P., McCornack, S. A., Morrison, K., & Park, H. S. (2014). Expertise in deception detection involves actively prompting diagnostic information rather than passive behavioral observation. *Human Communication Research, 40*(4), 442–462. https://doi.org/10.1111/hcre.12032

Levine, T. R., Kim, R. K., & Hamel, L. M. (2010). People lie for a reason: Three experiments documenting the principle of veracity. *Communication Research Reports, 27*(4), 271–285. https://doi.org/10.1080/08824096.2010.496334

Levine, T. R., McCornack, S. A., & Avery, P. B. (1992). Sex differences in emotional reactions to discovered deception. *Communication Quarterly, 40*(3), 289–296. https://doi.org/10.1080/01463379209369843

Levine, T. R., Serota, K. B., Carey, F., & Messer, D. (2013). Teenagers lie a lot: A further investigation into the prevalence of lying. *Communication Research Reports, 30*(3), 211–220. https://doi.org/10.1080/08824096.2013.806254

Lippard, P. V. (1988). "Ask me no questions, I'll tell you no lies": Situational exigencies for interpersonal deception. *Western Journal of Speech Communication, 52*(1), 91–103.

Littrell, S., Risko, E. F., & Fugelsang, J. A. (2021). The Bullshitting Frequency Scale: Development and psychometric properties. *British Journal of Social Psychology, 60*(1), 248–270. https://doi.org/10.1111/bjso.12379

Lobel, T. E., & Levanon, L. (1988). Self-esteem, need for approval, and cheating behavior in children. *Journal of Educational Psychology, 80*(1), 122–123. https://doi.org/10.1037/0022-0663.80.1.122

Lundquist, T., Ellingsen, T., Gribbe, E., & Johannesson, M. (2009). The aversion to lying. *Journal of Economic Behavior & Organization, 70*(1-2), 81–92. https://doi.org/10.1016/j.jebo.2009.02.010

Lykken, D. T. (1957). A study of anxiety in the sociopathic personality. *Journal of Abnormal and Clinical Psychology, 55*(1), 6–10. https://doi.org/10.1037/h0047232

Lykken, D. T. (1978). The psychopath and the lie detector. *Psychophysiology, 15*(2), 137–142. https://doi.org/10.1111/j.1469-8986.1978.tb01349.x

Lyons, M., & Jonason, P. K. (2015). Dark triad, tramps, and thieves: Psychopathy predicts a diverse range of theft-related attitudes and behaviors. *Journal of Individual Differences, 36*(4), 215–220. https://doi.org/10.1027/1614-0001/a000177

Mahon, J. E. (2008). Two definitions of lying. *The International Journal of Applied Philosophy*, *22*(2), 211–230. https://doi.org/10.5840/ijap200822216

Mandy, W. P. L., Skuse, D. H., Charman, T., & Frazier, T. W. (2012). In defense of lumping (and splitting). *Journal of the American Academy of Child & Adolescent Psychiatry*, *51*(4), 441–442. https://doi.org/10.1016/j.jaac.2012.02.004

Mann, H., Garcia-Rada, X., Houser, D., & Ariely, D. (2014). Everybody else is doing it: Exploring social transmission of lying behavior. *PLOS ONE*, *9*(10), e109591. https://doi.org/10.1371/journal.pone.0109591

Markowitz, D. M., & Levine, T. R. (2021). It's the situation and your disposition: A test of two honesty hypotheses. *Social Psychological and Personality Science*, *12*(2), 213–224. https://doi.org/10.1177/1948550619898976

Mauf, S., Martinez, R. M., Thali, M. J., & Bartsch, C. (2015). Made up by makeup—A case report about an exceptional kind of self-inflicted "injuries." *Forensic Science International*, *257*, e32–e37. https://doi.org/10.1016/j.forsciint.2015.10.027

Mazar, N., Amir, O., & Ariely, D. (2008). The dishonesty of honest people: A theory of self-concept maintenance. *JMR Journal of Marketing Research*, *45*(6), 633–644. https://doi.org/10.1509/jmkr.45.6.633

McCornack, S. A., Morrison, K., Paik, J. E., Wisner, A. M., & Zhu, X. (2014). Information manipulation theory 2: A propositional theory of deceptive discourse production. *Journal of Language and Social Psychology*, *33*(4), 348–377. https://doi.org/10.1177/0261927X14534656

McGlone, M., & Knapp, M. (2019). Historical perspectives on the study of lying and deception. In T. Docan-Morgan (Ed.), *The Palgrave handbook of deceptive communication* (pp. 3–28). Palgrave Macmillan.

Meehl, P. E. (1954). *Clinical versus statistical prediction: A theoretical analysis and a review of the evidence.* University of Minnesota Press. https://doi.org/10.1037/11281-000

Meijer, E. H., & Verschuere, B. (2015). The polygraph: Current practice and new approaches. In P. A. Granhag, A. Vrij, & B. Verschuere (Eds.), *Detecting deception: Current challenges and cognitive approaches* (pp. 59–80). Wiley-Blackwell.

Melin, G., Somers, K., Thanarajasingam, G., Couser, G., & Reese, M. (2008). A reverend's tale: Too tragic to be true? *Current Psychiatry*, *7*(5), 110.

Meropi, P., Bikos, C., & George, Z. (2018). Outlier detection in skewed data. *Simulation Modelling Practice and Theory*, *87*, 191–209. https://doi.org/10.1016/j.simpat.2018.05.010

Merriam-Webster. (2021). *Pathos.* https://www.merriam-webster.com/dictionary/pathos

Millon, T., Grossman, S., & Millon, C. (2015). *Manual for the MCMI-IV.* Pearson Assessments.

Mischel, W. (1968). *Personality and assessment*. Wiley.

Mitchell, D., & Francis, J. P. (2003). A case of factitious disorder presenting as alcohol dependence. *Substance Abuse, 24*(3), 187–189. https://doi.org/10.1080/08897070309511547

Modell, J. G., Mountz, J. M., & Ford, C. V. (1992). Pathological lying associated with thalamic dysfunction demonstrated by [99mTc]HMPAO SPECT. *The Journal of Neuropsychiatry and Clinical Neurosciences, 4*(4), 442–446. https://doi.org/10.1176/jnp.4.4.442

Mohtashemi, M., & Mui, L. (2003). Evolution of indirect reciprocity by social information: The role of trust and reputation in evolution of altruism. *Journal of Theoretical Biology, 223*(4), 523–531. https://doi.org/10.1016/S0022-5193(03)00143-7

Moon, J. W., Krems, J. A., & Cohen, A. B. (2018). Religious people are trusted because they are viewed as slow life-history strategists. *Psychological Science, 29*(6), 947–960. https://doi.org/10.1177/0956797617753606

Morey, L. C. (1996). *An interpretative guide to the Personality Assessment Inventory (PAI)*. Psychological Assessment Resources.

Mosby. (2017). *Mosby's pocket dictionary of medicine, nursing & health professions* (8th ed.). Mosby.

Moshagen, M., Musch, J., Ostapczuk, M., & Zhao, Z. (2010). Reducing socially desirable responses in epidemiologic surveys: An extension of the randomized-response technique. *Epidemiology, 21*(3), 379–382. https://doi.org/10.1097/EDE.0b013e3181d61dbc

Mukundan, C. R., Sumit, S., & Chetan, S. M. (2017). Brain electrical oscillations signature profiling (BEOS) for measuring the process of remembrance. *EC Neurology 8*(6), 217–230. https://www.ecronicon.com/ecne/pdf/ECNE-08-00256.pdf

Muzinic, L., Kozaric-Kovacic, D., & Marinic, I. (2016). Psychiatric aspects of normal and pathological lying. *International Journal of Law and Psychiatry, 46*, 88–93. https://doi.org/10.1016/j.ijlp.2016.02.036

National Research Council. (2003). *The polygraph and lie detection*. National Academies Press.

Newman, C. F., & Strauss, J. L. (2003). When clients are untruthful: Implications for the therapeutic alliance, case conceptualization, and intervention. *Journal of Cognitive Psychotherapy, 17*(3), 241–252. https://doi.org/10.1891/jcop.17.3.241.52534

Newmark, N., Adityanjee, & Kay, J. (1999). Pseudologia fantastica and factitious disorder: Review of the literature and a case report. *Comprehensive Psychiatry, 40*(2), 89–95. https://doi.org/10.1016/S0010-440X(99)90111-6

Ning, S. R., & Crossman, A. M. (2007). We believe in being honest: Examining subcultural differences in the acceptability of deception. *Journal of Applied Social Psychology, 37*(9), 2130–2155. https://doi.org/10.1111/j.1559-1816.2007.00254.x

Nolen-Hoeksema, S. (2007). *Lecture 18. What happens when things go wrong: Mental illness, Part I* [Guest Lecture by Professor Susan Nolen-Hoeksema]. https://oyc.yale.edu/psychology/psyc-110/lecture-18

Nolen-Hoeksema, S. (2011). *Abnormal psychology* (5th ed.). McGraw-Hill.

O'Grady, C. (2021, August 24). Fraudulent data raise questions about superstar honesty researcher: Dan Ariely denies fabricating data, but can't produce records to clear his name. *Science.* https://www.science.org/content/article/fraudulent-data-set-raise-questions-about-superstar-honesty-researcher

Oliveira, C. M., & Levine, T. R. (2008). Lie acceptability: A construct and measure. *Communication Research Reports, 25*(4), 282–288. https://doi.org/10.1080/08824090802440170

Olsen, D. P. (2012). Ethical issues: Putting the meds in the applesauce. *The American Journal of Nursing, 112*(3), 67–69. https://doi.org/10.1097/01.NAJ.0000412642.93516.42

Palmieri, J. J., & Stern, T. A. (2009). Lies in the doctor–patient relationship. *Primary Care Companion to the Journal of Clinical Psychiatry, 11*(4), 163–168. https://doi.org/10.4088/PCC.09r00780

Pankratz, L. (1998). *Patients who deceive: Assessment and management of risk in providing health care and financial benefits.* Charles C Thomas Publisher.

Pareto, V. (1896). *Cours d'economie politique* [Political economy course]. F. Rouge Libraire Editeur.

Park, H. S., Levine, T. R., McCornack, S. A., Morrison, K., & Ferrara, M. (2002). How people really detect lies. *Communication Monographs, 69*(2), 144–157. https://doi.org/10.1080/714041710

Park, H. S., Serota, K. B., & Levine, T. R. (2021). In search of Korean Outliars: "A few prolific liars" in South Korea. *Communication Research Reports, 38*(3), 206–215. https://doi.org/10.1080/08824096.2021.1922374

Patrick, C. J., & Iacono, W. G. (1989). Psychopathy, threat, and polygraph test accuracy. *Journal of Applied Psychology, 74*(2), 347–355. https://doi.org/10.1037/0021-9010.74.2.347

Patterson, J., & Kim, P. (1991). *The day America told the truth: What people really believe about everything that really matters.* Prentice Hall Press.

Paul Ekman Group, LLC. (2014). *Paul Ekman Group.* https://www.paulekman.com/

Paulhus, D. L., & Williams, K. M. (2002). The dark triad of personality: Narcissism, Machiavellianism and psychopathy. *Journal of Research in Personality, 36*(6), 556–563. https://doi.org/10.1016/S0092-6566(02)00505-6

Pauls, C. A., & Crost, N. W. (2005). Cognitive ability and self-reported efficacy of self-presentation predict faking on personality measures. *Journal of Individual Differences, 26*(4), 194–206. https://doi.org/10.1027/1614-0001.26.4.194

Pavlov, I. P. (1960). *Conditioned reflex: An investigation of the physiological activity of the cerebral cortex.* Dover Publications.

Pennebaker, J. W., Booth, R. J., Boyd, R. L., & Francis, M. E. (2015). *Linguistic Inquiry and Word Count: LIWC2015.* Pennebaker Conglomerates.

Pennisi, E. (2009). Origins. On the origin of cooperation. *Science, 325*(5945), 1196–1199. https://doi.org/10.1126/science.325_1196

Peters, S. (1876). *The True-blue Laws of Connecticut and New Haven and the False Blue-laws Invented by the Rev. Samuel Peters, to which are Added Specimens of the Laws and Judicial Proceedings of Other Colonies and Some Blue-laws of England in the Reign of James I.* American Publishing Company.

Peterson, C. (1996). Deception in intimate relationships. *International Journal of Psychology, 31*(6), 279–288. https://doi.org/10.1080/002075996401034

Peterson, J. (2017, May 5). *Side effects of telling lies* [Video]. YouTube. https://www.youtube.com/watch?v=23gRI_j5InA

Piff, P. K., Stancato, D. M., Côté, S., Mendoza-Denton, R., & Keltner, D. (2012). Higher social class predicts increased unethical behavior. *Proceedings of the National Academy of Sciences of the United States of America, 109*(11), 4086–4091. https://doi.org/10.1073/pnas.1118373109

Pinel, P. (1801). *Traité médico-philosophique sur l'aliénation mentale ou la manie* [Medico-philosophical treatise on insanity or mania]. Richard, Caille & Ravier.

Pinel, P. (1813). Nosographie philosophique [Philosophical nosography]. *Edinburgh Medical and Surgical Journal, 9*(34), 242–251.

Pitt, E., & Pitt, B. (1984). Cardiopathica fantastica. *American Heart Journal, 108*(1), 137–141. https://doi.org/10.1016/0002-8703(84)90556-8

Ponciano, J. (2020). Jeff Bezos becomes the first person ever worth $200 billion. *Forbes.* https://www.forbes.com/sites/jonathanponciano/2020/08/26/worlds-richest-billionaire-jeff-bezos-first-200-billion/?sh=7ce8c8994db7

Powell, G. E., Gudjonsson, G. H., & Mullen, P. (1983). Application of the guilty-knowledge technique in a case of pseudologia fantastica. *Personality and Individual Differences, 4*(2), 141–146. https://doi.org/10.1016/0191-8869(83)90013-2

Raskin, D. C., & Hare, R. D. (1978). Psychopathy and detection of deception in a prison population. *Psychophysiology, 15*(2), 126–136. https://doi.org/10.1111/j.1469-8986.1978.tb01348.x

Raspe, R. E. (2013). *Surprising adventures of Baron Munchausen.* https://www.gutenberg.org/files/3154/3154-h/3154-h.htm

Reid, J. (1947). A revised questioning technique in lie-detection tests. *Journal of Criminal Law and Criminology, 37*(6), 542–547. https://doi.org/10.2307/1138979

Risch, B. (1908). Ueber die phantastische Form des degenerativen Irrseins, Pseudologia phantastica [About the fantastic form of degenerative insanity, pseudologia phantastica]. *Allgemeine Zeitschrift fur Psychiatrie, 65*, 576–639.

Rogers, R. (2018). An introduction to response styles. In R. Rogers & S. D. Bender (Eds.), *Clinical assessment of malingering and deception* (4th ed., pp. 3–17). Guilford Press.

Rogers, R., & Bender, S. D. (2018). *Clinical assessment of malingering and deception* (4th ed.). Guilford Press.

Rogers, R., Sewell, K. W., & Gillard, N. D. (2010). *Structured interview of reported symptoms 2nd Edition: Professional manual.* Psychological Assessment Resources. https://doi.org/10.1002/9780470479216.corpsy0957

Rosenberg, M. (1965). *Society and the adolescent self-image.* Princeton University Press. https://doi.org/10.1515/9781400876136

Rosenhan, D. L. (1973). On being sane in insane places. *Science, 179*(4070), 250–258. https://doi.org/10.1126/science.179.4070.250

Sade, R. M. (2012). Why physicians should not lie for their patients. *American Journal of Bioethics, 12*(3), 17–19. https://doi.org/10.1080/15265161.2012.656800

Sarzyńska, J., Falkiewicz, M., Riegel, M., Babula, J., Margulies, D. S., Nęcka, E., Grabowska, A., & Szatkowska, I. (2017). More intelligent extraverts are more likely to deceive. *PLOS ONE, 12*(4), e0176591. https://doi.org/10.1371/journal.pone.0176591

Satel, S., & Lilienfeld, S. O. (2013). *Brainwashed: The seductive appeal of mindless neuroscience.* Basic Books.

Schein, C., & Gray, K. (2018). The theory of dyadic morality: Reinventing moral judgment by redefining harm. *Personality and Social Psychology Review, 22*(1), 32–70. https://doi.org/10.1177/1088868317698288

Schulz, F., & Grunow, D. (2012). Comparing diary and survey estimates on time use. *European Sociological Review, 28*(5), 622–632. https://doi.org/10.1093/esr/jcr030

Schweitzer, M. E., Hershey, J. C., & Bradlow, E. T. (2006). Promises and lies: Restoring violated trust. *Organizational Behavior and Human Decision Processes, 101*(1), 1–19. https://doi.org/10.1016/j.obhdp.2006.05.005

Selling, L. S. (1942). The psychiatric aspects of the pathological liar. *Nervous Child, 1*, 358–388.

Serota, K. B., & Levine, T. B. (2015). A few prolific liars: Variation in the prevalence of lying. *Journal of Language and Social Psychology, 34*(2), 138–157. https://doi.org/10.1177/0261927X14528804

Serota, K. B., Levine, T. R., & Boster, F. J. (2010). The prevalence of lying in America: Three studies of self-reported lies. *Human Communication Research*, *36*(1), 2–25. https://doi.org/10.1111/j.1468-2958.2009.01366.x

Shalvi, S., & Leiser, D. (2013). Moral firmness. *Journal of Economic Behavior & Organization*, *93*, 400–407. https://doi.org/10.1016/j.jebo.2013.03.014

Sharrock, R., & Cresswell, M. (1989). Pseudologia fantastica: A case study of a man charged with murder. *Medicine, Science, and the Law*, *29*(4), 323–328. https://doi.org/10.1177/002580248902900412

Simpson, G. G. (1945). The principles of classification and a classification of mammals. *Bulletin of the AMNH, Vol. 85*. American Museum of Natural History.

Skinner, B. F. (1938). *The behavior of organisms: An experimental analysis*. D. Appleton-Century Company.

Smith, D. L. (2004). *Why we lie: The evolutionary roots of deception and the unconscious mind*. St. Martin's Press.

Sodian, B. (1991). The development of deception in young children. *British Journal of Developmental Psychology*, *9*(1), 173–188. https://doi.org/10.1111/j.2044-835X.1991.tb00869.x

Sodian, B., & Frith, U. (1992). Deception and sabotage in autistic, retarded and normal children. *Child Psychology & Psychiatry & Allied Disciplines*, *33*(3), 591–605. https://doi.org/10.1111/j.1469-7610.1992.tb00893.x

Spence, S. A. (2005). Prefrontal white matter—The tissue of lies? Invited commentary on . . . Prefrontal white matter in pathological liars. *The British Journal of Psychiatry*, *187*(4), 326–327. https://doi.org/10.1192/bjp.187.4.326

Spurk, D., Keller, A. C., & Hirschi, A. (2016). Do bad guys get ahead or fall behind? Relationships of the dark triad of personality with objective and subjective career success. *Social Psychological & Personality Science*, *7*(2), 113–121. https://doi.org/10.1177/1948550615609735

Stemmermann, A. (1906). *Beitrage und Kasuistik der Pseudologia phantastica* [Contributions and casuistry of the pseudologia phantastica] in Healy, W., & Healy, M. T. (1915). Pathological lying, accusation and swindling. *Criminal Science Monographs*, *1*, 1–278.

Stephens-Davidowitz, S. (2017). *Everybody lies: Big data, new data, and what the internet can tell us about who we really are*. HarperCollins Publishers.

Stones, M. J. (1976). A study of a pathological liar. *Social Behavior and Personality*, *4*(2), 219–224. https://doi.org/10.2224/sbp.1976.4.2.219

Suchotzki, K., Verschuere, B., Van Bockstaele, B., Ben-Shakhar, G., & Crombez, G. (2017). Lying takes time: A meta-analysis on reaction time measures of deception. *Psychological Bulletin*, *143*(4), 428–453. https://doi.org/10.1037/bul0000087

Swartz, C. M. (2003). Clinical controversies. Pseudomania. *The Psychiatric Times, 20*(6), 23–25.

Talwar, V., & Crossman, A. (2011). From little white lies to filthy liars: The evolution of honesty and deception in young children. *Advances in Child Development and Behavior, 40*, 139–179. https://doi.org/10.1016/B978-0-12-386491-8.00004-9

Talwar, V., Lavoie, J., & Crossman, A. M. (2019). Carving Pinocchio: Longitudinal examination of children's lying for different goals. *Journal of Experimental Child Psychology, 181*, 34–55. https://doi.org/10.1016/j.jecp.2018.12.003

Talwar, V., & Lee, K. (2002a). Development of lying to conceal a transgression: Children's control of expressive behaviour during verbal deception. *International Journal of Behavioral Development, 26*(5), 436–444. https://doi.org/10.1080/01650250143000373

Talwar, V., & Lee, K. (2002b). Emergence of white lie-telling in children between 3 and 7 years of age. *Merrill-Palmer Quarterly, 48*(2), 160–181. https://doi.org/10.1353/mpq.2002.0009

Talwar, V., Murphy, S. M., & Lee, K. (2007). White lie-telling in children for politeness purposes. *International Journal of Behavioral Development, 31*(1), 1–11. https://doi.org/10.1177/0165025406073530

Tangney, J. P., Stuewig, J., & Mashek, D. J. (2007). Moral emotions and moral behavior. *Annual Review of Psychology, 58*(1), 345–372. https://doi.org/10.1146/annurev.psych.56.091103.070145

Tavaglione, N., & Hurst, S. A. (2012). Why physicians ought to lie for their patients. *The American Journal of Bioethics, 12*(3), 4–12. https://doi.org/10.1080/15265161.2011.652797

Teasdale, K., & Kent, G. (1995). The use of deception in nursing. *Journal of Medical Ethics, 21*(2), 77–81. https://doi.org/10.1136/jme.21.2.77

Thom, R., Teslyar, P., & Friedman, R. (2017). Pseudologia fantastica in the emergency department: A case report and review of the literature. *Case Reports in Psychiatry*, article ID 8961256. https://doi.org/10.1155/2017/8961256

Tomaszewski, M. (2021). *"My pet died" (& other lies to get out of work): 2021 study.* https://zety.com/blog/excuses-to-get-out-of-work

Treanor, K. E. (2012). *Defining, understanding and diagnosing pathological lying (pseudologia fantastica): An empirical and theoretical investigation into what constitutes pathological lying* [Doctoral dissertation]. University of Wollongong, Australia. https://ro.uow.edu.au/cgi/viewcontent.cgi?article=4817&context=theses

Tugaleva, V. (2013, October 11). Lessons from a former liar: The power of owning our stories. *Tiny Buddha*. Retrieved July 7, 2022, from https://tinybuddha.com/blog/lessons-former-liar-power-owning-stories/

Tukey, J. W. (1977). *Exploratory data analysis*. Pearson.

Vedantam, S. (Host). (2018, April 9). Everybody lies, and that's not always a bad thing [Audio podcast episode]. *Hidden brain*. NPR. https://www.npr.org/2018/04/09/599930273/everybody-lies-and-thats-not-always-a-bad-thing

Verigin, B. L., Meijer, E. H., Bogaard, G., & Vrij, A. (2019). Lie prevalence, lie characteristics and strategies of self-reported good liars. *PLOS ONE, 14*(12), e0225566. https://doi.org/10.1371/journal.pone.0225566

Verschuere, B., Crombez, G., Koster, E. H. W., & Uzieblo, K. (2006). Psychopathy and physiological detection of concealed information: A review. *Psychologica Belgica, 46*(1-2), 99–116. https://doi.org/10.5334/pb-46-1-2-99

Verschuere, B., Meijer, E. H., Jim, A., Hoogesteyn, K., Orthey, R., McCarthy, R. J., Skowronski, J. J., Acar, O. A., Aczel, B., Bakos, B. E., Barbosa, F., Baskin, E., Bègue, L., Ben-Shakhar, G., Birt, A. R., Blatz, L., Charman, S. D., Claesen, A., Clay, S. L., . . . Yıldız, E. (2018). Registered Replication Report on Mazar, Amir, and Ariely (2008). *Advances in Methods and Practices in Psychological Science, 1*(3), 299–317. https://doi.org/10.1177/2515245918781032

Vésteinsdóttir, V., Joinson, A., Reips, U. D., Danielsdottir, H. B., Thorarinsdottir, E. A., & Thorsdottir, F. (2019). Questions on honest responding. *Behavior Research Methods, 51*(2), 811–825. https://doi.org/10.3758/s13428-018-1121-9

Vrij, A. (2000). *Detecting lies and deceit: The psychology of lying and the implications for professional practice*. John Wiley & Sons.

Vrij, A. (2008). *Detecting lies and deceit: Pitfalls and opportunities* (2nd ed.). John Wiley & Sons.

Vrij, A. (2015). Verbal lie detection tools: Statement validity analysis, reality monitoring and scientific content analysis. In P. A. Granhag, A. Vrij, & B. Verschuere (Eds.), *Detecting deception: Current challenges and cognitive approaches* (pp. 3–35). Wiley-Blackwell.

Vrij, A., Fisher, R. P., & Blank, H. (2017). A cognitive approach to lie detection: A meta-analysis. *Legal and Criminological Psychology, 22*(1), 1–21. https://doi.org/10.1111/lcrp.12088

Vrij, A., Fisher, R., Mann, S., & Leal, S. (2006). Detecting deception by manipulating cognitive load. *Trends in Cognitive Sciences, 10*(4), 141–142. https://doi.org/10.1016/j.tics.2006.02.003

Vrij, A., Fisher, R., Mann, S., & Leal, S. (2008). A cognitive load approach to lie detection. *Journal of Investigative Psychology and Offender Profiling, 5*(1-2), 39–43. https://doi.org/10.1002/jip.82

Vrij, A., Granhag, P. A., Mann, S., & Leal, S. (2011). Outsmarting the liars: Toward a cognitive lie detection approach. *Current Directions in Psychological Science, 20*(1), 28–32. https://doi.org/10.1177/0963721410391245

Vrij, A., Granhag, P. A., & Porter, S. (2010). Pitfalls and opportunities in non-verbal and verbal lie detection. *Psychological Science in the Public Interest,* *11*(3), 89–121. https://doi.org/10.1177/1529100610390861

Vrij, A., Hartwig, M., & Granhag, P. A. (2019). Reading lies: Nonverbal communication and deception. *Annual Review of Psychology, 70*(1), 295–317. https://doi.org/10.1146/annurev-psych-010418-103135

Vrij, A., & Mann, S. (2006). Criteria-based content analysis: An empirical test of its underlying processes. *Psychology, Crime & Law, 12*(4), 337–349. https://doi.org/10.1080/10683160500129007

Vrij, A., Meissner, C. A., & Kassin, S. M. (2015). Problems in expert deception detection and the risk of false confessions: No proof to the contrary in Levine et al. (2014). *Psychology, Crime & Law, 21*(9), 901–909. https://doi.org/10.1080/1068316X.2015.1054389

Ward, D. A. (1986). Self-esteem and dishonest behavior revisited. *The Journal of Social Psychology, 126*(6), 709–713. https://doi.org/10.1080/00224545.1986.9713652

Warmelink, L. (2021). *Lying across the lifespan* [Webinar]. Deception Research Society. https://www.youtube.com/watch?v=6SkgzpJHHX8

Wharton, F. (1868). *A treatise on the criminal law of the United States (6th ed.): Vol. 1. Pleading and evidence.* Kay & Bro.

Whitty, M. T., & Carville, S. E. (2008). Would I lie to you? Self-serving lies and other-oriented lies told across different media. *Computers in Human Behavior, 24*(3), 1021–1031. https://doi.org/10.1016/j.chb.2007.03.004

Wiersma, D. (1933). On pathological lying. *Character and Personality, 2*(1), 48–61. https://doi.org/10.1111/j.1467-6494.1933.tb02081.x

Williams, S., Moore, K., Crossman, A. M., & Talwar, V. (2016). The role of executive functions and theory of mind in children's prosocial lie-telling. *Journal of Experimental Child Psychology, 141,* 256–266. https://doi.org/10.1016/j.jecp.2015.08.001

Williams, S. M., Kirmayer, M., Simon, T., & Talwar, V. (2013). Children's antisocial and prosocial lies to familiar and unfamiliar adults. *Infant and Child Development, 22*(4), 430–438. https://doi.org/10.1002/icd.1802

Wind, Y., & Lerner, D. (1979). On the measurement of purchase data: Surveys versus purchase diaries. *JMR, Journal of Marketing Research, 16*(1), 39–47. https://doi.org/10.1177/002224377901600106

World Health Organization. (1992). *The ICD-10 classification of mental and behavioural disorders: Clinical descriptions and diagnostic guidelines.*

World Health Organization. (2019). *International statistical classification of diseases and related health problems* (11th ed.). https://icd.who.int/

World Health Organization. (2021a). *Classification of diseases (ICD)*. https:// www.who.int/standards/classifications/classification-of-diseases

World Health Organization. (2021b). *History of the development of the* ICD. https://cdn.who.int/media/docs/default-source/classification/icd/historyoficd. pdf?sfvrsn=b9e617af_3&download=true

World Health Organization. (2021c). ICD-11 *fact sheet.* https://icd.who.int/en/ docs/icd11factsheet_en.pdf

Wright, G. R. T., Berry, C. J., & Bird, G. (2013). Deceptively simple . . . The "deception-general" ability and the need to put the liar under the spotlight. *Frontiers in Neuroscience, 7,* 152. https://doi.org/10.3389/fnins.2013.00152

Yalom, I. D., & Leszcz, M. (2020). *The theory and practice of group psychotherapy* (6th ed.). Basic.

Yang, Y., Raine, A., Lencz, T., Bihrle, S., Lacasse, L., & Colletti, P. (2005). Prefrontal white matter in pathological liars. *The British Journal of Psychiatry, 187*(4), 320–325. https://doi.org/10.1192/bjp.187.4.320

Yang, Y., Raine, A., Narr, K. L., Lencz, T., LaCasse, L., Colletti, P., & Toga, A. W. (2007). Localisation of increased prefrontal white matter in pathological liars. *The British Journal of Psychiatry, 190*(2), 174–175. https://doi.org/10.1192/ bjp.bp.106.025056

Yip, J. A., & Schweitzer, M. E. (2016). Mad and misleading: Incidental anger promotes deception. *Organizational Behavior and Human Decision Processes, 137,* 207–217. https://doi.org/10.1016/j.obhdp.2016.09.006

Yu, J. (2009, Fall–Winter). The compulsive liar apologizes to her therapist for certain fabrications and omissions. *TriQuarterly, 135–136,* 461–462.

Zhong, C. B., Bohns, V. K., & Gino, F. (2010). Good lamps are the best police: Darkness increases dishonesty and self-interested behavior. *Psychological Science, 21*(3), 311–314. https://doi.org/10.1177/0956797609360754

Zvi, L., & Elaad, E. (2018). Correlates of narcissism, self-reported lies, and self-assessed abilities to tell and detect lies, tell truths, and believe others. *Journal of Investigative Psychology and Offender Profiling, 15*(3), 271–286. https:// doi.org/10.1002/jip.1511

Index

About the Authors

Drew A. Curtis, PhD, is a licensed psychologist, Rodgers Distinguished Faculty, and the director of the PsyD and MS counseling psychology programs at Angelo State University (ASU). He is the past-president for the Southwestern Psychological Association and currently serves as the president for Psychological Association of Greater West Texas. Dr. Curtis has taught a variety of courses for more than 15 years, primarily teaching abnormal psychology, psychopathology, and deception. He established and oversees the Clinical Science and Deception lab at ASU. His research has specifically focused on pathological lying and deception in the context of therapy, within health care professions, intimate relationships, and parental relationships. Dr. Curtis has presented on a theoretical basis for understanding pathological lying and has collaborated with Dr. Hart on several research studies examining pathological lying. Other research has examined psychomythology of psychopathology and teaching of psychology. He has published an abnormal psychology textbook, a book about psychopathology, several papers on deception, and received various research grants and awards for his research. He is also coauthor of another book with Dr. Hart, the forthcoming *Big Liars: How Pathological and Compulsive Deceivers Hurt, Gaslight, and Exasperate Everyone Around Them.*

Christian L. Hart, PhD, is a professor of psychology and director of the psychological science graduate program at Texas Woman's University. He holds an MS and PhD in experimental psychology and has been a professor for almost 20 years. He teaches courses in deception and forensic psychology and conducts research primarily on lying and deception. He is also the former president and current executive director of the Southwestern Psychological Association. Before becoming a professor, Dr. Hart held the rank of lieutenant commander in the U.S. Navy, where he served as an aerospace experimental psychologist and taught at the Navy Test Pilot School. He is coauthor of the forthcoming book *Big Liars: How Pathological and Compulsive Deceivers Hurt, Gaslight, and Exasperate Everyone Around Them.*